MAKE AMERICA HEALTHY AGAIN

Lessons from a 50 Year Surgical Odyssey

CHARLES ANTINORI MD, FACS

Copyright © 2025 Charles Antinori MD, FACS.

All rights reserved. No part of this book may be reproduced, stored, or transmitted by any means—whether auditory, graphic, mechanical, or electronic—without written permission of both publisher and author, except in the case of brief excerpts used in critical articles and reviews. Unauthorized reproduction of any part of this work is illegal and is punishable by law.

ISBN: 979-8-89419-607-7 (sc)
ISBN: 979-8-89419-608-4 (hc)
ISBN: 979-8-89419-609-1 (e)

Because of the dynamic nature of the Internet, any web addresses or links contained in this book may have changed since publication and may no longer be valid. The views expressed in this work are solely those of the author and do not necessarily reflect the views of the publisher, and the publisher hereby disclaims any responsibility for them.

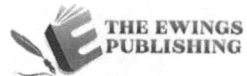

One Galleria Blvd., Suite 1900, Metairie, LA 70001
(504) 702-6708

To Chaz and Alessa, my Muse.

CONTENTS

Acknowledgements vii

Preface ix

Introduction xi

Chapter 1   CYA 1

Chapter 2   Surgical Training 9

Chapter 3   How to Improve the Health Care System 14

Chapter 4   Electronic Health Records 20

Chapter 5   HIPAA and Medical Records 24

Chapter 6   The Operating Room 28

Chapter 7   The Rise and Fall of American Medicine 34

Chapter 8   Dr. DeBakey Stories 40

Chapter 9   Some Technological Advances 49

Chapter 10   Easy Steps to Better Health for America 62

Epilogue 87

Bibliography 89

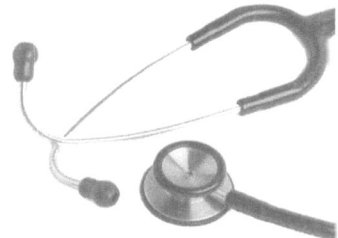

ACKNOWLEDGEMENTS

I would like to thank my daughter, Alessa, for her help and encouragement. My sister, Marilyn Depice, and friends Christine Rothwell and Olga Russial for their technical assistance. My office managers, Nilsa Larriu-Mazzeo and Ginni McCarty for all their help over the years. Finally, my family and of course my mother, Elizabeth, for everything.

I hope I did not forget anyone but I probably did.

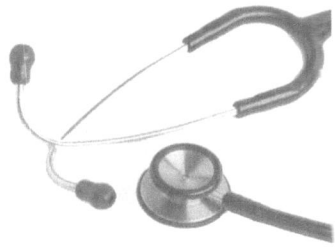

PREFACE

I would just like to point out that it took me about a year and a half to write this book which was first published in May of 2024. During that whole time, I had a Make America Great Again hat sitting on my model of the human heart right next to my computer screen as seen in the accompanying photograph. I rarely wore the hat because I live in New Jersey and anything MAGA could provoke hostile reactions. Actually I live in Cape May, NJ which is fairly conservative area even though NJ is a deep blue state. However, it is a resort town and for most of the year there are a lot of tourists in town from liberal Democratic strongholds like New York City, North Jersey and Philadelphia. My five-year-old granddaughter got a lesson in politics when we had to take down my Trump/VanDrew sign because she was running a lemonade stand in front of my house and several of her customers complained about it. This also started a small argument between her mother and her brother, my son, who felt strongly that we should not take the sign down. Emotions ran high around this election even in a close-knit family!

By the way, my granddaughter made an astonishing $603 that day on the lemonade stand! She even took Venmo! I mention all of this because I want my readers to know that I picked the title for the book around February 2024 which was long before President Trump and Robert F. Kennedy, Jr. started using the slogan "Make America Healthy Again". I was working away at the computer and looking at the MAGA hat and the idea just struck me that "Make America Healthy Again" would be a good catchy title.

I hope you enjoy the book. It is an easy read. It is even more topical now due to the tragic murder of the United Healthcare CEO. This has stimulated a lot of discussion about what is wrong with the American healthcare system.

—CHA

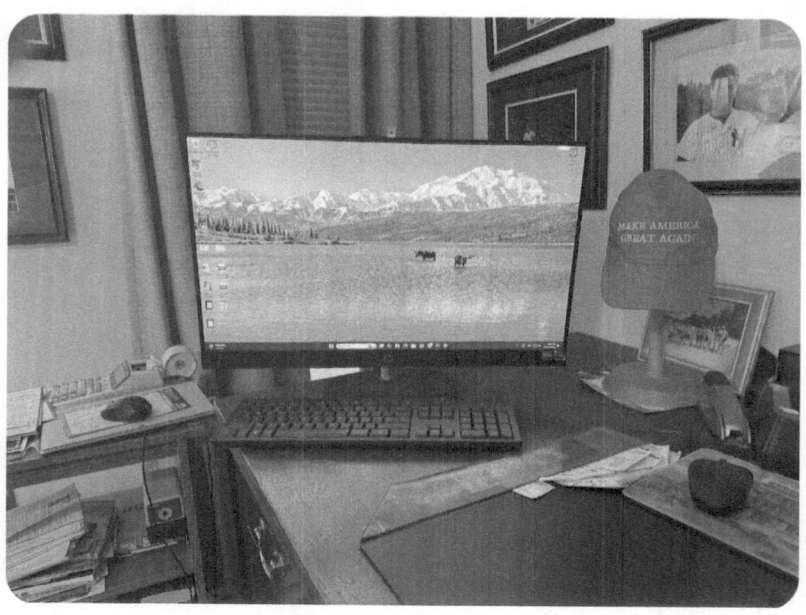

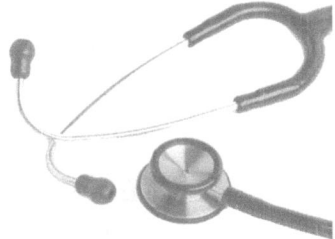

INTRODUCTION

As my late friend, Charles Krauthammer, MD, often mentions in his book, *Things That Matter*, "Medicine is a very satisfying field" Surgery is even more satisfying than other areas of medicine because it is so 'hands on.' The surgeon-patient relationship is extremely close. Almost all surgical patients do well and are extremely grateful. This makes the work very rewarding."[1]

However, things can go wrong, and medicine can become stressful at times. When I interviewed for a thoracic surgical residency at the University of Alabama with Dr. John Kirklin, a legendary heart surgeon, he told me, "Cardiac surgery had the highest highs and the lowest lows." Truer words have never been spoken. The occasional bad outcome can be very distressing even if it does not result in malpractice litigation.

The cost of medical education is rising exponentially, and the time required for training continues to increase. There are four years of expensive medical school after college. Then residency and fellowship training can extend from three to ten years. In the surgical fields, it is rarely less than five years. Due to changes in reimbursement and a

---

[1] Charles Krauthammer, MD, *Things That Matter*

rise in the number of employed physicians in practice, the financial rewards are diminishing.

Although physicians only receive about 20 percent of health care spending, costs continue to rise nearing 20 percent of the gross domestic product. More and better diagnostic procedures arrive almost every day. There are also better medications and innovative new surgical procedures such as the use of robots. Generally, this improves care, but it always drives up costs.

In this book, I will discuss all these factors in detail. I will also relate some of the personal stories that have made my last fifty years interesting and largely enjoyable. I will make some suggestions for improving the health care delivery system in our country. Finally, I will make some simple suggestions that would make all us Americans healthy again.

CHAPTER 1

CYA

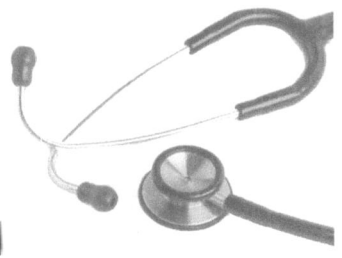

If we want to have a national health care system, the first thing we should do is pass a constitutional amendment. We need to do this for a variety of reasons.

Firstly, virtually everyone in the United States thinks we already have a right to health care. I'm pretty sure our forefathers would have put this in the Bill of Rights if health care had existed when they wrote the Constitution. The medical historians I have read suggest that it wasn't until around 1925 that the average patient had a better-than-average chance of benefiting from an encounter with a physician. That makes sense. It wasn't until the late nineteenth century that Pasteur and Semmelweis developed the germ theory—how microorganisms relate to disease. In the early 1900s, thyroid hormone, insulin, and blood typing became available. Before that, going to the doctor was a crapshoot. If you watch the old cowboy movies, you'll see that all the doctors seem to do was tell people to boil water and get clean sheets. Then they always went in and pulled out that old bullet as if it was the lead in the bullet that was going to kill the patient.

Secondly, all you have to do is go to any emergency room in the United States and you'll see people walking in expecting the best possible medical care independent of their ability to pay. Fortunately, up to this point, they've been able to get it. However, for a variety of factors including increasing human longevity and the proliferation of sophisticated medical knowledge and equipment, costs have been increasing exponentially. Providing the best possible medical care is using up a tremendous percentage of our gross national product.

Personally, I have never seen anyone denied any needed medical care, and I've been involved in the health care system since 1969 in some of the poorest cities in the country like Camden, New Jersey. In fact, if anything, I think people often get too much medical care. This is partly because there are so many sophisticated tests available and largely because health care providers' fear of litigation for missing something forces doctors to order so many tests. Tests beget tests. Findings on one test necessitate another test to verify those findings. Then the second test suggests further testing and so on. Right now, this is delivering state-of-the-art medical care, but it is extremely expensive. Our politicians and economists are concerned because medical care is consuming nearly 20 percent of the gross domestic product.

A constitutional amendment would help to clear the path for tort reform. President George W. Bush was talking about having national tort reform legislation before 9/11 came along and scuttled that discussion. I had already read that, if a national tort reform act was passed, there would be legal challenges that would likely be successful because the right to health care is not guaranteed by the Constitution but the right to sue is. The only significant savings available in this health care system now would be through tort reform. Eliminating "futile care" is estimated to save about 10 percent, but deciding what is futile is difficult. Right now, if you try to "pull the plug" on Grandma because you think her situation is futile, you leave yourself wide open for a lawsuit if the family thinks she might have made it through. Living wills have not helped much because, no matter what Grandma stipulated in her living will, it's the family that doctors have to deal with when she is obtunded. It's the family members who sue after she dies.

Most of these suits don't go anywhere, but from the malpractice insurer's point of view, it's a "hit" on that doctor. They haven't got the time or interest to get into the right or wrong of the issue. If they have to pay a lawyer to meet with the doctor even once to go over the case, it's a black mark on that doctor's record. It's just about the money.

This hasn't changed during my entire career. When I was a surgical intern at Columbia Presbyterian in New York in 1973, we did head trauma evaluations. We evaluated any person who came in who had bumped his head. Often a mother would come in with a little baby and say something like, "I wasn't watching for a few minutes. I think he might have fallen." We would do a quick but thorough neurological evaluation. Then we would usually give the parents something called a "head sheet," which told them what to do and what to watch out for in the child. This was good, cost-effective medicine. However, we could not blast the patients out of the emergency room without getting skull films. This was before the days of computed tomography scans (CT scans). There was an article lying in one of the drawers in the emergency room that reported that 10,000 skull films had not shown one unsuspected skull fracture. This was a virtually totally useless test.

Skull films at that time cost about $65. I made about $50 for working a twenty-four-hour shift in the emergency room. On the average day, I might order five or ten sets of useless skull films. For some reason, people, particularly people in the legal system, believe in the mystical power of X-rays over the good clinical judgment and physical examination of physicians. This is about the only reason I can come up with for ordering skull films, and this goes for an awful lot of other tests as well.

I once had this conversation with my program director when I was an intern, explaining my views just as I have here. Do you know what he told me? "Get the skull films!" This logic system has not changed at all in over forty years, but the tests have gotten more sophisticated and more expensive.

Like every other surgeon, I pay a large amount of money every year for malpractice insurance. This is a significant expense comprising approximately 15 to 20 percent of my gross earnings. However, the amount is peanuts in terms of how much money could be saved with tort reform. The big saving would be in the ability to not have to order that extra test just to rule out the one last possible diagnosis. If we could go back to a system something like the system that was in place in the 1970s and 1980s where sophisticated tests were available when needed but not expected to be done in every single case, we would save a lot of money.

The fact that so much of our medical care is delivered through the emergency room system is also inefficient and wasteful. Probably only something like 10 to 20 percent of cases seen in the emergency room are truly emergencies. People just go to the emergency room because it's more convenient than making an appointment with the family physician. Indigent patients make up approximately 20 percent of the population in the areas where I have worked in New Jersey. These people use the emergency room because they know they will get care before they have to pay for it. Often the charges they incur are never paid for at all. When an insurance company balks at doing an expensive sophisticated test in an effort to try to control medical costs, many doctors simply tell the patient to go to the emergency room where they will just get the test done without going through the approval process.

Just today, as I was sitting down to write this, I was called by an emergency room provider about an indigent Spanish-speaking patient who had gallstones. She had no fever, no white count, no jaundice, and no other signs of severe illness. We admitted her because she had been seen in the emergency room a week earlier with exactly the same picture but had not taken the antibiotics that had been recommended and had not scheduled an outpatient appointment to set up cholecystectomy. Now she'll sit in the hospital for a day or two until we can take out her gallbladder. This is a huge waste of resources. We are spending more money on those who put the least into the system. We do this because it is the compassionate thing to do, but it's getting to the point where our country just cannot afford this type of care.

I pay a lot for health insurance, but I tell my children not to go to the emergency room unless t is absolutely necessary and to clear it with me first! As soon as they step foot in the emergency room, I end up with about $500 worth of bills from deductibles, copays, and other charges. Also, I have to take hours out of my day between 9:00 am and 4:00 pm to call the various billing companies to sort out what I'm actually supposed to pay. When my daughter drove her car into a guard rail along the New Jersey Garden State Parkway, I found out that the Parkway bills anyone who causes damage. Then she had to take a one-mile, $500 ambulance ride to the emergency room even though she wasn't hurt because she was under eighteen. It's a state law. I could see where that might be a good idea sometimes, but since it's New Jersey, I'm sure the ambulance lobbyists had something to do with that one.

The liability situation also affects emergency room doctors. If it were up to them, anyone with any remote possibility of being sick would be admitted to the hospital because then their job is done. Any liability shifts to the admitting physicians and consultants. You can't blame them. It's human nature to CYA (cover your ass).

Another way the emergency room drives up costs is repeated testing. I've already related the story about how I was forced to do useless $65 skull films when I was an intern from 1973 to 1974. Now when a patient walks into an emergency room, he is very likely to get a CT scan, and the real cost of this is probably over $500. My son received a bill for $ 3,000 for a CT scan, but that's another story. Marty Makary, MD, devotes several chapters in his book, *The Price We Pay: What Broke American Health Care—and How to Fix It*, to the vast differences in amounts paid by patients for emergency room visits, lab tests, ambulance rides, and especially helicopter rides.

Most CT scans are ordered on a computer using a drop-down menu, so the only information the radiologist gets is "abdominal pain" or "fever" or something brief like that. Because the radiologist who reads the films has to cover himself, he must include every possible diagnosis he can see in his analysis of the image and often throws in phrases like "can't rule out appendicitis" or "clinical correlation required." Often, to further cover themselves, they throw in a sentence at the end like "if more information needed consider an MRI." The emergency room doctor reads this and often feels he needs to order the MRI (magnetic resonance imaging) to cover himself. It goes on and on. The real cost of an MRI is probably over one thousand dollars. It's not unusual for me to see a consult in the emergency room on a patient who has had five or six CT scans in the space of a few months.

I have one patient who is on Medicaid. He had an extensive laparotomy (open abdominal exploration) years ago at a trauma center for a gunshot wound. Since then, he has had about six more laparotomies for abdominal pain due to bowel obstruction caused by adhesions from the previous surgery. We have not had to operate on him for several years now. However, every time he comes into the emergency room, which is often, the providers have to order a CT scan. He actually had nineteen CT scans in a six-month period. There were times when he had two in a week. We are all paying for this! Not only that, but blood work was repeated. He was seen by the emergency room doctors who often consulted me. Sometimes he got admitted to the hospitalists. This situation just kept perpetuating itself.

It's paradoxical—the more you pay for health insurance, the more you demonstrate that you can pay. So, if you have insurance, you get hit with co-pays, deductibles, and other charges. If you don't pay anything for health care, there is no barrier to going to the emergency room to have even the most trivial symptoms and issues checked out.

There are a lot of paradoxical situations in our current health care system. You must read *Catch 22* by Joseph Heller to understand it and maintain your sanity. For example, prisoners typically have great health care plans. Doctors who operate on a patient who is currently incarcerated usually get paid fairly well. The day after the prisoners are released, they find themselves with no health care coverage.

Another paradoxical thing is that the more serious the condition a doctor treats, the more that doctor is morally obligated to provide that treatment for free. Therefore, the less our system feels the doctor must be reimbursed. Dentists get paid more for a root canal than a surgeon might get paid for a thoracotomy. Similarly, doctors who've provide cosmetic and less essential services like plastic surgeons and dermatologists can charge more for their services then a surgeon covering the emergency room who gets called in to do an emergency appendectomy or cholecystectomy.

The most highly sought residencies now are not neurosurgery or thoracic surgery or any of the other fields that were traditionally prestigious. Today's graduates gravitate to fields in which they will have a schedule; do shift work, and rarely get called in for an emergency.

CHAPTER 2

SURGICAL TRAINING

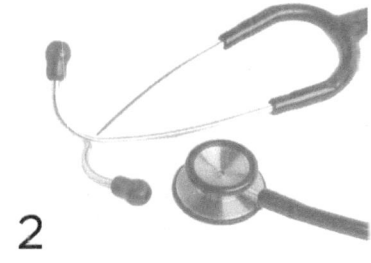

I don't know if many people realize how difficult it is to become a surgeon. At present, doctors to be must finish college and then go on to four years of medical school. After that, there's residency. General surgery residencies usually run about five years now. Many times, residents take fellowships afterwards for another year or two to subspecialize.

For example, after finishing Regis High School in New York City, I went to Cornell University for three years. After that, I did two years at Dartmouth Medical School, which was a two-year school at that time. I transferred to Harvard Medical School to finish medical training. After that, I did five years of general surgery residency at New York–Presbyterian/Columbia University. I finished my training with a two-year residency with Dr. DeBakey at Baylor College of Medicine in Houston. I was very lucky that I got to finish my residency with a four-month rotation in Saudi Arabia doing heart surgery.

Nowadays, that education would cost over several hundred thousand dollars. Cornell could be easily $50,000 a year; the four years of medical school could be another $50,000 a year. Residents now generally make about $50,000 a year for working eighty hours a week. After the Libby Zion case in New York City, the work hours have been reduced to 80 hours a week. We worked 100 to 110 hours a week when we were "on call" every third night and 120 to 130 hours a week when we were on every other night. There are only 168 hours in the week, and we had to sleep sometime. That schedule didn't provide much time for family or recreation.

Surgical residencies are a lot like Marine boot camp except Marine boot camp lasts seven or eight weeks while surgical residencies last seven or eight years. There's probably not as much intense physical activity for doctors as there is for soldiers, but there are long hours that are definitely physically demanding, and there is a tremendous amount of mental stress. One good thing it is that it prepares doctors to work hard when they finally get out in practice. My partners and I used to joke that we worked only half days—twelve hours!

What worries me now is not the reduction in the work hours, although there are problems there that I will discuss. I'm most concerned that every one of the surgical residents in our program is approximately $300,000 in debt. These are extremely intelligent, extremely hard-working young men and women who are now in their early thirties. They don't own homes or much else, and they continue to work very hard for eighty hours a week.

People think that this is not going to be a problem because they will make so much money when they go into practice. This is no longer true. They will be very lucky to start out at $200,000 a year, and if present trends continue, this will likely peak at about $350,000 a year. They will pay at least a third of that in taxes. In that situation, it will take a very long time to pay off $300,000 of debt. Remember, they don't own homes yet; they just have big mortgages!

I have followed baseball very closely all my life, particularly the New York Yankees. In 1990, Don Mattingly was the highest-paid New

York Yankee. He was the captain of the team, and he made about three million dollars a year. Other top ballplayers like Tim Raines at that time made about the same. A very busy surgeon at that time—a neurosurgeon, a cardiovascular surgeon, a plastic surgeon, an orthopedic surgeon—could possibly make a million dollars a year. This didn't occur very often. I never made that amount, but a few people did. Everything had to be working right, and the surgeon had to be extremely busy. He had to have a good payer mix, a good deal with his hospital, good partners, and a lot of luck. Most of all, he had to work very hard for twelve months a year.

So, at that time, the ratio from top ballplayer to top surgeon was about 3 to 1. Fast-forward to the present, and that same surgeon has a difficult time earning even $500,000 in 2023 dollars. This would be about $250,000 in 1990 dollars. I just read the other day that the average Major League baseball player now makes four million dollars a year. There are several top earners making thirty million a year. So now the ratio in thirty-three years has gone from 3 to 1 to about 60 to 1. I don't begrudge the ballplayers a nickel of that money. They are extremely talented and have relatively short careers; however, you have to wonder about the priorities of a society that allows this sort of drastic change to occur.

If present trends continue, it's bound to get worse. Just a few years ago, both houses of Congress finally agreed to get rid of the dreaded "sustainable growth rate." This mechanism was used to grind down physician reimbursement for more than twenty years. During that time, the average payment of Social Security benefits has gone up 52 percent. This is basically a low-end cost-of-living increase designed to keep our retirees above the poverty level. For the same period of time, physician reimbursement has gone up 5 percent. This means that physicians lost about 47 percent of the cost of living over the last twenty years or so. This fits very well with the perception of most physicians. Furthermore, as I've said, it's going to get worse.

Getting rid of the sustainable growth rate was considered a huge victory by organized medicine. As part of the deal, physicians got a 0.5 percent raise every year for the next five years. The cost of living for this period continued to increase at about 4 percent a year (pre the Biden administration). So, physicians lost another 15 to 20 percent in buying power. How can you expect the best and the brightest to continue going into the system?

I have a friend who was a nurse. She worked in the neonatal intensive care unit in one of the large hospitals in Philadelphia. She was making over $100,000 a year working three twelve-hour shifts a week in the Baylor system. She decided to go to medical school while still working as a nurse. She is a hard worker! Despite continuing to earn her nurse's income, she ended up about $250,000 in debt. She is now in the middle of a five-year residency making $50,000 a year. She will be over forty when she finishes residency.

A smart kid can graduate from college at age twenty-one and from business school at twenty-three or law school at twenty-five and start making money with minimal debt. Why would that same kid want to go to medical school and do six to seven years of residency to start earning money at age thirty or thirty-five with $300,000 in debt. Remember also that these doctors will be working eighty hours a week on call every third or fourth night during their twenties when other professionals are working more reasonable hours, starting families, and having fun.

Something else that strikes me as unfair now is that most of the student loans were at 7 percent interest when mortgages were running 3 to 4 percent. I get a report from Harvard Medical School every year, and the most interesting number in it for me is the average debt of the graduating student. It's been about $110,000 to $120,000 recently. Most of the time, a resident doesn't make enough money to pay off even the interest during residency, so by the time he finishes residency five to eight years later, $110,000 of debt could easily have risen to $200,000. Harvard is one of the most well-endowed private medical schools, so it's likely that most students come out with even more debt from other schools. Perhaps students going to state schools come out with a little bit less. Students more and more are electing to go to less prestigious state schools even if they are accepted at schools like Harvard Med because they don't want to come out with crippling debt.

The concern I have about the shortening of the residence work week to eighty hours is not that I resent current doctors working less than we did. It's that they are getting only four-fifths of the experience that we got because we worked at least an average of a hundred hours a week to their eighty. They see in five years what we saw in four.

To make things worse, there is a lot more to learn than there was when I trained. For example, I had to learn only one way to do an appendix or gallbladder surgery, which was open with an old-fashioned incision. Now there are three methods residents must learn—open, laparoscopic, and robotic, and there is less time for learning. Aside from the technical aspect, there is a lot more research and literature residents must study. This is part of the reason that many of the current residents feel they need a fellowship for additional training.

Fellowships, however, are a bit of a double-edged sword. Doctors do get more training, but it's generally more subspecialized, and doctors emerge years older and deeper in debt. Most of the fellowships train the residents in a few specific procedures, which gets them further away from the "bread-and-butter surgery" that they are likely to see when they go into practice. It's difficult for doctors to come straight out of residency or fellowship and do complex procedures like open-heart surgery or transplants. They just don't have the experience, and very few practitioners will refer to them.

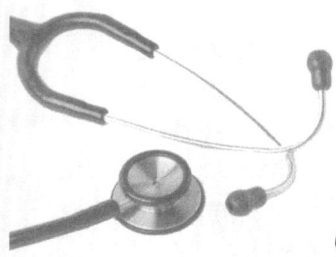

CHAPTER 3

HOW TO IMPROVE THE HEALTH CARE SYSTEM

As I said in the first chapter, the first thing we need to do is pass a constitutional amendment that guarantees health care a right of every American citizen. This makes sense only because everyone in the United States already feels that he or she has a right to good health care, and everyone has received excellent health care to this point.

The advantage of such a constitutional amendment is that we could limit litigation. This is the only significant savings available in the present health care system. Also, the amendment would have to spell out some guidelines about what can be expected from the citizens and from the health care system. The details would have to be left to the individual states, but I think that there should be some mention of the rational use of limited health care resources. We all hate the word *rationing*, but I think we must understand that we have to follow a practice of "rational use."

If I were designing the health care system, I would designate a single payer, and that would have to be the federal government.

For the first forty-five years of my life, I would never have said that, but over the last twenty years, it's become increasingly apparent to me that this is the only possible solution. However, rather than the hodgepodge system that we have now that includes Medicare, Medicaid, the Affordable Care Act, and private insurers, I would start all over with a clean sheet of paper.

I think I would leave Medicare much the same as it is and make Medicaid health insurance for the poor, and I mean a system that actually pays for services rendered. Then I would have the federal government supply what I call Major Medical. In this system, the government would start paying whenever a person's medical bills exceeded an established threshold, say $40,000. I'm certainly not wedded to the figure of $40,000. This is a number that would have to be worked out with a lot of accountants and underwriters from the insurance industry, but it certainly could be done. Whatever limit was set, people would be able to pursue different methods to achieve the insurance up to the point that "major medical" would kick in.

Using $40,000 as a threshold, wealthy people might not have to purchase any health insurance whatsoever; they could just pay the first $40,000 out of pocket and then the government would take over. Working down the economic ladder, most of the middle class would be able to purchase reasonably inexpensive insurance to cover up to the $40,000. It would be inexpensive because the insurer would have to worry only about liability up to $40,000. I would imagine that many times this premium would be paid by the patient's employer as it is often now. Essentially this would be a "private insurance pool." The existing system of health savings accounts could also cover this. Then some threshold of income insurance would be provided for the poor people as it is now with Medicaid. I am not enough of an accountant to tell you exactly what be the income limit below which you would get federal insurance or exactly what would be the threshold where the major medical would kick in. These numbers could be computed and then adjusted on a yearly basis.

While we are talking about reconstructing the entire health care system, I would strongly suggest that, rather than have malpractice cases haggled out in court in front of people who by and large have no idea what's being discussed, they could be handled by an insurance panel. You know the old saying—You don't get tried by a jury of your peers; you get tried by a jury of people who couldn't get out of jury duty.

A highly educated dedicated jury pool is exactly what plaintiff attorneys do not want. Medical issues are still so sophisticated that the topics and issues that are discussed in malpractice cases cannot be fairly adjudicated by any lay audience in most cases.

The Workmen's Compensation system has been in place for many years and works reasonably well. Numerous studies over the years have shown that malpractice litigation could much more easily and more efficiently be handled by a panel of experts from all the involved fields much like the Workmen's Compensation panels. It would be necessary to have doctors, lawyers, and insurance experts on the panel. When a person suffered a negative medical outcome, the panel could do the math. They could figure out how much the negative result would cost the person for the rest of his life and make some sort of fair payment without necessarily assigning guilt or innocence to any parties involved in the situation.

The problem with the situation now is that the cost of all the discovery, depositions, and litigation is greater in many cases than what the payout needs to be. This could all be handled as an insurance matter without the need to prove someone guilty or innocent. I would not try to tell you that there has never been malpractice committed in the United States, but I believe in my heart of hearts that there has never been deliberate malpractice committed. Unfortunately, the way the system works now, the only way for a plaintiff to get paid is to prove that doctors or hospitals are guilty of malpractice. When this happens, a huge chunk of the settlement goes to the legal team's fees and compensation.

Numerous studies have shown that the system can be handled much more efficiently as an insurance system. Eventually there would be standard payouts for standard occurrences. Doctors and hospitals could pay into the system in much the way they pay for malpractice insurance now. Possibly even patients could purchase insurance for individual operations just as people buy insurance for individual plane flights for a very small amount of money. Riskier procedures would require larger payments from the doctors and hospitals and possibly patients into the insurance pool. This could all be worked out in time by underwriters working fairly and honestly.

By the way, this will *never* happen because, unfortunately, just about every legislative body in this country at the local, state, and federal levels is comprised of at least 60 percent lawyers. They will never approve of any of this even though I think they know already that it would be the best thing for our country.

This type of liability is not only affecting medicine; it is also costing townships huge amounts of money when they get sued and run up huge legal fees that have to be distributed over relatively small numbers of households in the town. Small businesses are also suffering. A pipe burst in my house a few years ago, and the plumber and I were crawling around under my house on a cold February day trying to find a shut-off valve. He said to me that he thought he paid more malpractice insurance that I did. I won the bet, but I found out that he paid about $50,000 a year and actually stopped installing sprinkler systems because they were driving his liability up so much they weren't worth doing! This reminded me of orthopedic surgeons who stop doing spine surgery because the risk of litigation outweighs any amount of money they can make from the procedures. Other procedures have been abandoned for the same reason.

Another initiative that could improve the overall health of Americans would be better education about health. The average American gets a lot of information about healthy food choices from commercials made by the people selling the food; this is hardly an unbiased source. I was shocked when I read a book by Michael Greger, MD, and Gene Stone, MD, entitled *How Not to Die: Discover the Foods Scientifically Proven to Prevent and Reverse Disease*. They report that organizations like the American Dietetic Association are often voluntary organizations; that is, they depend on donations to survive. Some of the largest donors are soft drink manufacturers and members of the meat packing industry. It is difficult for associations to tell people that soda and red meat are bad health choices when they depend on these corporations for funding.

Robert F. Kennedy Jr. pointed out in his book, *The Real Anthony Fauci: Bill Gates, Big Pharma, and the Global War on Democracy and Public Health*, that medical journals, which I have always held as the last bastions of truth, are also sometimes compromised in reporting results because they have become dependent on the advertising revenue that comes from the big pharmaceutical corporations.

It would be challenging to implement, but I would totally revise the way "health" is being taught in primary and secondary schools in this country. A lot of basic, hard knowledge about health and nutrition is no longer controversial. A graduated course progressing through grades three through twelve could provide a solid background in basic human biology. It's not rocket science!

Health education could start with the introduction to the basic systems: circulatory, musculoskeletal, integumentary, endocrine, and so forth. Then progressively, lessons could fill in more detailed anatomy and physiology. Eventually, the plan could include information on proper nutrition and signs of common diseases. I think a little knowledge could prevent a lot of costly emergency room visits.

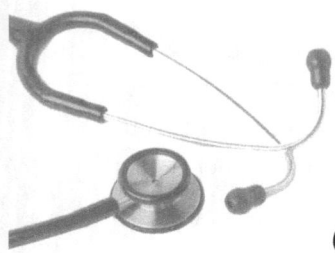

CHAPTER 4

ELECTRONIC HEALTH RECORDS

Government support of electronic health records started with George Bush Sr.'s administration with a small amount of money. This is all very well documented in Dr. Robert Wachter's excellent book on electronic health records, *The Digital Doctor: Hope, Hype, and Harm at the Dawn of Medicine's Computer Age.* During the Obama administration in 2009, the Health Information Technology for Economic and Clinical Health Act (HITECH Act) was passed. This essentially required doctors and hospitals to computerize by 2014.

In many ways, this was an improvement in medical care because, when the system is working properly, a physician can access a patient's medical records from almost anywhere as long as there is a computer (or other device) and an internet connection. Records are most commonly accessed from hospitals, doctors' offices, and doctors' homes.

Accessing patient records from home has been identified as one of the major causes of physician burnout. One of the problems is that the last two hours in the office often turn out to be late in the evening. Many times, doctors want to have dinner with their families, so they leave the office and take their laptops home. Then, after dinner at some point, they must sit down for a few hours to finish up their computer work. I would emphasize that this work must be done in a timely fashion; if doctors let too much time to go by, they are likely to make more mistakes.

Numerous studies have analyzed the effect that electronic health records (EHR) has had on physicians' time management. They have generally shown that physicians now spend about one-fourth of their office time face-to-face with patients. About half the time is spent on the computer, and the rest on administrative chores such as phone calls, meetings, and other obligations. The average primary care doctors spend about two hours doing work after they have seen their last patient of the day. Very often, they complete the work at home later in the evening, which leads to burnout.

As I have mentioned, computer systems, when they work properly, have generally improved medical care, but they have drawbacks.

1. Computers and software have increased costs tremendously. Generally speaking, the information technology (IT) departments in hospitals have become one of the largest and most expensive departments. As anyone who works with computers on a regular basis knows, they require constant maintenance, and there are frequent glitches.
2. No computer has even so much as placed a Band-Aid on a patient.
3. Computer software occasionally contributes to catastrophic mistakes; for example, in his book, *The Digital Doctor*, Dr. Robert Wachter devotes about a third of the text to an incident in which a pediatric patient was given thirty-six doses of an antibiotic through a series of minor errors between doctors, nurses, pharmacists, and computer

systems. The computer system involved was Epic Software, which is generally regarded as the best of the electronic health systems. Incidentally it is also the most expensive.

4. Almost every day now in the news there is an article about some hospital system or other corporate entity that has been hacked by an external source and forced to pay ransom to get the system running again. This probably happens more often than we know because many of the victims are embarrassed and simply pay the ransom without calling attention to the situation.

A day after I wrote the preceding paragraph, I received an email informing me that our local Federally Qualified Health care Association (FQHA) primary care group had been hacked. This is the type of facility that supplies most of the outpatient care to indigent patients. We were advised not to share any patient information with them until the issue is resolved.

Another problem with computer systems that Dr. Wachter raises in his book is getting the different systems to interface with one another. There are about three major computer systems and probably ten more minor systems that are being used around the country. I'm not a computer specialist, but I understand that it's very difficult to get them to speak to each other. In our section of New Jersey, an electronic Health Information Organization known as NJSHINE is working to promote the sharing of electronic health information, and sometimes it helps. However often even hospitals that are close geographically have different operating systems, and it's difficult to get them to interface. Also, since it's difficult, it costs money, and no one wants to pay to maintain an expensive system that's used only a few times a month.

Another complicated boondoggle involving medical computer systems is the billing systems; specifically, the International

Classification of Diseases (ICD) diagnostic codes and the Current Procedural Terminology (CPT) therapeutic codes. There were about 16,000 diagnostic codes in ICD-9, which had was replaced by ICD 10, which contains about 64,000 codes.

Whenever doctors perform a procedure, they must come up with a few of the 64,000 diagnostic codes to justify it. Like "appendicitis" for an appendectomy. That's an easy one, but even for an easy one, it might be necessary to add mitigating factors like obesity or diabetes. Every diagnosis has numerous subvariants too.

Then, after doctors get their diagnoses, they go to the Current Procedural Terminology book and add whatever procedures have been performed. Fortunately, so far, the CPT system has not been changed.

However, doctors must watch the fact that there are usually several possible names for whatever procedure they do; for example, gastrectomy, partial gastric resection, subtotal gastric resection, and so forth. Sometimes minor differences in the names of the procedures can lead to huge discrepancies in doctors' reimbursements.

This system is so complicated that, in a typical medical office, about 6 percent of gross income is spent on the billing process. This also illustrates the advantage of specialists like plastic surgeons who do not have to get involved with billing insurance companies or Medicare for cosmetic procedures. I won't even talk about billing Medicaid because that s an oxymoron. One of my office managers had worked for plastic surgeons at one point in time. She said that all they had to do for billing was to write on a sheet of paper "Facelift $3,600" and hand it to the patient. That's another benefit of doing elective non-emergency procedures.

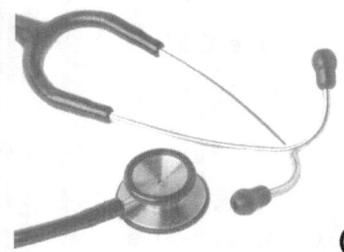

CHAPTER 5

HIPAA AND MEDICAL RECORDS

*No matter how cynical you get,
it is impossible to keep up with reality*
—Lily Tomlin

The Health Insurance Portability and Accountability Act of 1996 (HIPAA) is a federal law designed to protect sensitive patient health information from being disclosed without the patient's consent or knowledge. This is another example of a well-intentioned federal law that has caused all sorts of collateral damage and complications.

One of the simplest complications is that now, when a patient's family member calls and asks for information about a patient, doctors and staff members must check to make sure that the caller is on the list of patient-approved contacts before they can disclose information. This takes time. Besides that, if the patient didn't include a particular relative on the list and providers can't answer questions, many times, callers become quite upset, which can damage the doctor-patient relationship.

Another consequence of this is that numerous trees have been sacrificed to generate all the paper necessary to send out notices every month outlining the various "privacy policies" of every institution with which doctors are involved. I must get at least six or seven of these statements a month, and they all go immediately into the recycling bin.

Furthermore, these companies generate an entire industry involved in encrypted text messaging. The cynical side of me thinks that these companies were started by the brothers-in-law of the legislators that pushed HIPPA through.

Anyway, like most people, physicians have found that texting is an extremely rapid and convenient way of communicating with each other. If nothing else, it saves "small-talk time" when the goal is to just relay a single message. It also has the advantage of being a permanent record so the receiver can review it at his or her leisure and respond as needed. Since it's typed, it's generally readable, and detailed names, numbers, and dates can be included. Unfortunately, the normal text messaging that we do on the typical iPhone or Android is not encrypted; therefore, it is not HIPAA compliant; therefore, sending patient information via a text message from an iPhone could be a HIPAA violation and engender fines up to $50,000. I don't know anyone who has ever had to pay that, but I've heard that it has happened. Most of us still text back and forth and just limit the amount of information we include.

Typically, if I want a call back about a patient having some abdominal pain I might text "call me re-GB in room 333." Personally, I don't see how this reveals any sensitive information, but the folks who made this law seem to think it does. Therefore, companies have come up with complicated systems to encrypt text messaging. These systems seem to fascinate the administrators of the health care system. I guess it's because they don't want to get any HIPPA penalties, which would be a black eye on their record. These encryption systems are extremely cumbersome and sometimes dangerous. One that we used for a while was annoying because it sent the alert through an electronic channel that was separate from the one used to send the message. So, when we got an alert on our phones, we'd get our phones out, but the message would not be there yet. To make matters worse, sometimes it could take days for the message to show up. Sometimes it didn't show up at all.

To remedy this, developers kept updating the system and making it more complicated. The last time I put an update into my phone, it jammed up my phone so badly that I couldn't make or receive any calls. Sometimes I feel that we have forgotten that the primary function of a phone is still to make and receive calls!

We just started using a new system that I have not installed yet. Maybe it's because the residents and nurses who are using it absolutely hate it. Apparently, even make a simple call is complicated and cumbersome. Again, this is against the backdrop of text messaging, which is used dozens if not hundreds of times a day with absolutely no problem. I'm not aware of any horrible leaks of patient information from this practice.

Another bit of craziness that we endure on a daily basis as physicians is signing medical records. This is a ridiculous system designed purely to link doctors to orders so that, when a lawsuit comes up, it's easier to identify the doctors involved.

I have been saying this for decades: We cannot not sign the orders because they have already been executed!

Doctors also must sign because their admitting and/or operating privileges might be suspended if they are delinquent. In other fields, I believe it's called restraint of trade if people are forced to do something under the threat of losing their means of making a living!

Years ago, when we had paper charts, we had to go down to medical records in the hospital for about an hour every week and manually, with an actual pen, sign our names or initials hundreds of times. We could not dispute the documents because, for example, the drug that had been ordered had been given weeks before. Or the test had been done weeks ago. So, we just signed our names.

This was one thing that got a little better when we went to computer systems. Now, whenever we sign on to our electronic health record system, a list comes up of "Orders to be Cosigned." These were entered by residents and have been executed by nurses and other staff members already. I have had as many as two hundred orders come up when I'm busy. On average, it's probably thirty to fifty a day. All doctors have to do is click "Select all," which highlights all the orders. With one more click—"Approve"—they all disappear. No one could possibly read them all! Also, there's no point in reading them since they have already been executed!

I remember speaking to the vice president of medical affairs at Cooper Hospital in Camden, New Jersey, sometime around 1999 when the hospital had first put in a computerized system. She told me this was how we were going to sign the orders. I said to her, "But, Doctor, we won't even be looking at them!" She said, "Do you look at them now?" She was right. No one looked at them; we just signed away as fast as we could!

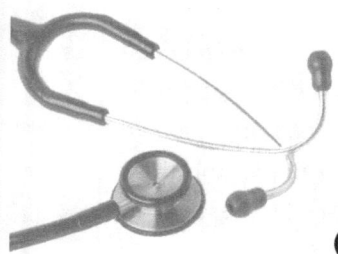

CHAPTER 6

THE OPERATING ROOM

Res ipse loquitor

Obviously, the operating room is the heart and soul of surgery. It's amazing how it's changed over the fifty years I've been in practice, and changes have almost completely been for the better.

Every little thing has improved. When I started my medical practice in 1973, the mortality rate for patients who received anesthesia was one in about 4,000; today it is something like one in 100,000. That means that one patient out of every 4,000 or so used to die simply from being put to sleep. Probably the most common cause of these deaths has been the intubating of the esophagus instead of the trachea, where it is supposed to go. Most people wonder how that could possibly happen, but it's surprisingly easy to do.

Intubating is placing a breathing tube into the patient's trachea. However, the trachea is right in front of the esophagus and actually harder to get into than the esophagus. So, years ago, occasionally, the breathing tube would be put in the esophagus. The oxygen and other gases that were given would be pumped into the stomach instead of the lungs. When this happened, patients would often have what is known as a "code" or cardiac arrest because the lungs were not delivering oxygen to the blood stream, which was not delivering oxygen to the heart. So the heart would stop beating. Most of the time, the patient would survive, albeit possibly with a stroke or some other serious injury. Occasionally they would expire.

Technology has improved tremendously in this area. Now, we monitor all patients by hooking them up to an electrocardiogram (EKG) machine. We also monitor them by pulse oxygenation, which indicates how much oxygen is being delivered to the bloodstream. Probably most importantly, we measure expired carbon dioxide. If you are alive, you have to be producing carbon dioxide. In the operating room, if the monitoring device indicates no expired carbon dioxide, the anesthesiologist knows something is wrong, and whatever it is can usually be fixed promptly.

These are just a few of probably hundreds of small, incremental improvements that have been made in technique that have drastically reduced the dangers of surgery. We have better antibiotics and better antibiotic guidelines. There are better anesthetic gases and drugs. In general, the doctors, nurses, and nurse anesthetists who do the work are better educated and more attuned to avoiding problems.

A pumping device on the patient's calf muscles during surgery can prevent the formation of clots, which cuts down on the number of pulmonary emboli experienced by patients overall. There is also much better perioperative use of anticoagulation to cut down on pulmonary emboli, which can be a sudden, lethal postoperative complication.

Extra corporeal membrane oxygenation (ECMO) can be used to oxygenate a patient while his heart or lungs are not functioning.

This previously was used primarily in small children, but now it is used more commonly in adults. This is, in many ways, similar to the heart-lung machine, but the heart-lung machine can be used only for a few hours before it starts to cause significant complications. ECMO can be used for days.

There are a few things that have not improved. For example, when I started out, most physicians and surgeons hired qualified nurses to work in their offices. These were generally either registered nurses (RNs) or licensed professional nurses (LPNs). The RN received more training than the LPN. Now the RN degree has almost been replaced by the bachelor of nursing (BSN).

Nurses now do a four-year college program and get a bachelor's degree in nursing. Previously there were local programs based in hospitals. The nursing students went to school in the hospital and had on-the-job training. Both systems worked well in turning out excellent, compassionate, knowledgeable nurses. The bachelor programs generally turn out nurses with more "book knowledge." The other programs were stronger on the day-to-day bedside nursing.

The problem doctors face now involves decreased reimbursement and the rise in the cost of running an office. Nurses' salaries, which are not terribly high, have become too expensive. One solution is to use "medical assistants" (MAs) where appropriate. These are generally nice, young, well-motivated people, but their training involves only about six months after high school. Many go directly into this field after high school. Many also come to it after trying different jobs such as working at Burger King.

Suffice it to say that the overall level of knowledge that can be infused in this type of program compared to a four-year nursing program is limited. Some of these people work hard, and in time, they become excellent at their job. On the other hand, many of them who are intelligent realize how limited their field is and how low their salary is. Often, they go on to nursing school or even medical school.

The MAs who are not so good, unfortunately, tend to stay on the job; that is, unless they get a better offer from McDonald's or Burger King. Pregnancies and childcare also make scheduling somewhat chaotic for female employees. This, from the doctor's point of view, makes the entire office practice much more difficult to manage.

Something similar has happened in the operating room. When I started out, we worked with surgical nurses, also known as scrub nurses. These were fully trained registered nurses who wanted to work in the operating room. Most of them made a career out of this specialty. In fact, we still have nurses in the OR, but their average age now is somewhere in the mid to late fifties. Also, they have been slightly pushed aside and asked to do a job that is more complicated but, in my view, not as interesting as scrubbing in the OR. Most of the registered nurses in the OR now generally perform a job that is known as "circulating."

Circulating was always a complicated job. Essentially it could be described as a very high-level "go fetch." They had to track down all the equipment that the surgeons needed—sutures, tools, instruments, and other devices. When computers came along, the job got even more complicated. Now they not only had to go fetch items, but they also had to document each one in the computer. Speaking for myself, I would probably go crazy if I tried to do this job. Anyway, this job requires the talents of fully trained registered scrub nurse.

To fill the void created by making the registered nurses into circulators, a field was created that is known as "scrub techs." These are dedicated people who actually scrub on all the cases. This generally requires several years of training and at least six months of experience. They get very good at scrubbing because they do it day in day out. However, a big part of their training and responsibilities is to make sure that the "counts" are all correct. This is a drawn-out process. At the start of an operation, the scrub tech and the circulating nurse count the instruments that are on the OR table, and there might be a hundred or more. All the sponges, all the little knife blades, needles, and any other thing that could possibly be left inside the patient is counted and documented. The scrub tech's primary responsibility is making sure that the counts are correct.

When I trained with Dr. DeBakey, he used to throw the needles on the floor when he was finished with them because that way they could not end up in the patient. This is a very good system, but it is total anathema to the system used everywhere else. Anyone training with him had to be very careful working anywhere else after spending a few months in his service. Throwing needles on the floor made people persona non grata in any other OR.

It is not necessary for scrub techs to have extensive medical training about actual medical conditions and why certain procedures are carried out; this information isn't necessary for them to do their jobs properly. This makes them somewhat less interested in following exactly what the surgeon is doing and more interested in making sure that the infernal counts come out right.

To refer again back to Dr. DeBakey, he worked with one scrub nurse who knew his routines as well as he did. The beauty of this is that she knew what instrument he was going to need, and he didn't even have to ask for it. This made the surgery flow much more smoothly. In long, complicated operations this was extremely important.

Scrub techs and even the nurses when they do scrub are less interested now in following the operation and are more interested in making sure everything is organized on their "back table," which is in the opposite direction from the surgeon. Therefore, they rarely watch what the surgeon is doing and are more interested in making sure that all the counts are going correctly.

By the way, in malpractice cases where an instrument or a device is left in the patient *the counts are invariably correct!* The legal phrase for this situation is *res ipsa loquitor,* Latin for "The thing speaks for itself." In other words, a doctor is not supposed to leave a clamp in the patient's abdomen no matter how complicated the surgery is!

Another problem in the system is that, to retain good help, it is important that nurses, techs, and other help get lunch breaks and other breaks. There is such a huge concern about making sure the counts come out correctly, but after all the checklists and routines that we go through to make sure that nothing is ever left the patient, the single biggest factor causing something to be left in the patient is a change in OR personnel during an operation. It has also clearly been demonstrated that changing personnel during an operation

increases the risk of patient infection. It stands to reason that the more people who walk in and out of the operating room while a patient's wound is open, the more likely there is to be an infection.

By the same reasoning, the more people who were involved in counting the instruments, sponges, needles, knife blades, and other items, the more chance there is for a miscount. When multiple lunch breaks and other breaks are taken, there is a higher chance for a miscount. Another factor is that, very often, the people who are doing the counting learned to count in different languages.

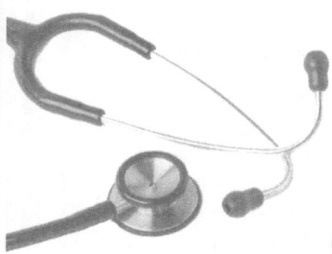

CHAPTER 7

THE RISE AND FALL OF AMERICAN MEDICINE

No good deed goes unpunished.

As I mentioned in the introduction, in the history of medicine, it was not until around 1925 that the average patient benefited from the average encounter with a physician. In the late 1800s Pasteur and Semmelweis developed the bacterial theory of disease. Roentgen developed X-rays. The Curies discovered radioactivity.

In the early 1900s, ABO and Rh blood typing developed, insulin came into use, and drugs such as digoxin and thyroid were available. Vaccines were developed for such killers as smallpox and typhus. In the 1920s, the sulfonamides—the first antibiotics—were developed. They were not very effective and were somewhat dangerous. In 1937, Fleming discovered penicillin, but it did not come into widespread use until after World War II. The circumstances of the war forced the mass production of penicillin, which made it widely available to everyone at a reasonable price. In the 1950s, Dr. Salk and Dr. Sabin developed vaccines for polio, which had previously been the scourge of the summers. The fact that they refused to make any profit from their discoveries was a huge public relations boon to the medical profession. All through the 1950s and 1960s, more antibiotics were developed; for example, tetracycline and erythromycin, the so-called "wonder drugs." It was a great time for medicine.

Next came the Great Society. Medicare was passed in 1964 and came into being around 1966. Doctors, through the American Medical Society (AMA) fought against this tooth and nail. They feared loss of control of their professions. They were prophets! However, for thirty years we thought they were crazy. Because the doctors fought so hard against Medicare, they managed to get a very good deal initially. Reimbursement was set at approximately the seventy-fifth percentile of "usual and customary fees." Suddenly, everyone over sixty-five years of age had good health insurance. This also happens to be the demographic group that is the most likely to get sick. Medicare ushered in a huge burgeoning of medical science.

Before 1965, physicians were hesitant to do major procedures on elderly patients for fear that, if something went wrong, the family would be bankrupted. I started my surgical residency at Columbia Presbyterian in New York City in 1973. There were still many surgeons there who had spent most of their careers practicing in the pre-Medicare era. We used to present every complication weekly at mortality and morbidity conference no matter how minor. Every time we presented a complication on an elderly patient who had a hernia or gallbladder done, one of the old surgeons would say, "Why did you do that operation on a seventy-year-old patient?"

It's interesting that Medicare was passed at a time when the country was in the midst of the Vietnam War just as Obamacare was passed during the wars in Afghanistan and Iraq; nevertheless, Medicare ushered in the golden period of American medicine. As I have said, I have never seen anyone refused any needed treatment whether there were on Medicare or not or whether they could pay or not.

Medical care improved every day in every way. We were able to do more and more complicated and advanced procedures. Indeed, procedures like open-heart surgery, which was first done in 1956 with the development of the heart-lung machine at Thomas Jefferson Hospital in Philadelphia, became commonplace by the end of the 1970s. In the 1980s, millions of coronary bypasses and valves were performed, and most of them were fully paid for by Medicare or commercial insurance.

Around 1990, folks at the Centers for Medicare and Medicaid Services (CMS) were running a huge budget that was getting bigger every year. With the pending aging of the baby boomer generation, the situation figured to get a lot worse. In 1992, the first cuts started going through Medicare. All through the 1990s, surgeons in particular were financially decimated, taking about a 10% cut every year until 2002 when the payment system was frozen for almost twenty years. Since 1996, the Social Security benefits that are tied to the cost-of-living index, have gone up over 50 percent while the average reimbursement to physicians has gone up 5 percent. The overhead in the medical profession in that period has probably gone up more than 50 percent spurred by huge increases in the cost of liability insurance and health insurance as well as general expenses.

Interestingly, in 1986, Medicare paid about $4,600 for a triple coronary artery bypass. This was the most common open-heart operation. In general, it involves opening the chest and putting the patient on cardiopulmonary bypass, which means a machine does the work of the patient's heart and lungs. Then three vessels are constructed that bypass blockages or severe narrowing of the native arteries. In 2023, Medicare reimbursed $2,400 in 2023 dollars. Factoring in inflation, this works out to be about one fourth of the 1986 reimbursement.

This means that, in 1986, if a cardiac surgeon did just a hundred triple coronary artery bypasses and nothing else on Medicare patients, he would gross about $460,000. I was practicing in New Jersey back then and can tell you that my malpractice insurance ran about $30,000 and all expenses including office, assistants, cars, phones, etc. ran about $100,000. That would leave about $360,000 1986 dollars in salary, which was a pretty good reimbursement.

Run the same equation for the same cardiac surgeon in 2023. A hundred triple bypasses for Medicare would generate about $240,000; however, malpractice and other expenses would have gone up to about $200,000 leaving $40,000, which is the average poverty level in America now.

Proportional decreases in reimbursement applies to almost all procedures. As I mentioned, simply freezing the reimbursement for almost twenty years starting in 2002 reduced the value by half at least.

This led to a lot of unlikely consequences. For one thing, cardiovascular surgery went from being one of the highest-paying and most-sought-after residencies to one of the least popular. It is not simply that surgeons are in it for the money; the work is very interesting and rewarding in itself. It's just that, after surgeons do one of the longest, most-grueling training programs and work the longest, most-unpredictable hours, they would like to be able to support themselves and their families at a level that's a bit above the poverty level.

An anecdote from personal experience illustrates my point. Around 2000, I was on "backup call" for the weekend. At this time, our group had two doctors on call: one to cover general surgery and one to cover cardiovascular surgery. Then we had one or two doctors on backup call in case the primary on-call person was overwhelmed or tied up in the OR all day. There was also a rule in New Jersey that two cardiac surgeons were required for an open-heart case— one as surgeon and one as assistant. This was a good rule because the surgery is long and complicated, and even with two surgeons working, it would generally take four to five hours to do a typical triple coronary bypass. Medicare paid the assistant 16 percent of the surgeon's fee.

At around eight o'clock on Friday evening, my partner, who was on primary call, alerted me that there was a patient in the cardiac catheterization lab, and the cardiologists were having a lot of trouble. He thought we were going to have to take the patient to the operating room. Now my night was set. I couldn't go out. I couldn't drink alcohol. It wasn't even worth renting a movie because there was a good chance I'd have to leave in the middle.

Sure enough, at around eleven that night, I was called again and went in to do the procedure. We started at about midnight and finished at around four in the morning, which made me tired all weekend. It was difficult to even sleep during the day because I kept getting calls.

For this, my reimbursement as assistant was 16 percent of about $2,400 or $384! I should tell you that this hospital was in Camden, New Jersey. The parking lot was across the street from the hospital, and people had been assaulted and even shot while crossing that street. After dark, security personnel had to walk nurses to the parking lot when their shift ended.

I never did this experiment, but I would bet that, if you randomly called people in the Camden suburbs like Cherry Hill or Haddonfield and asked them to come into Camden and cross the street by themselves in front of the hospital at eleven o'clock on a Friday night for $384, very few would do it! And that's without doing the four hours of open-heart surgery!

Another story like that involves a babysitter. This time I was on backup call for general surgery. It was a beautiful August Sunday afternoon. I was in the early stages of a divorce, and we had not worked out our schedule with the kids yet, so I had my children with me—my son, age seven, and my daughter, age five. (Incidentally, the divorce worked out well. The kids are fine, and my ex is one of my best friends.)

Since I was on backup call and had the kids, I had hired a babysitter to be backup for me! She was a great, well-educated girl who had been a full-time nanny for the kids for a few years. Also, she could drive and had a car. At around two in the afternoon on this beautiful Sunday, I was sitting next to our pool, and the kids were swimming; my partner called and told me he had to do an emergency colon resection on an obese patient and needed help. I called the babysitter and was waiting at the end of my driveway when she arrived. I drove to the hospital, helped with the colon resection, and helped my partner finish rounds. Altogether, I was gone for four hours.

I was paying the babysitter $2 per hour while she was on backup and $15 an hour while she was actually taking care of the kids, which came to $60 cash for the four hours. I would be reimbursed about 16 percent of $1,000 for assisting on the colon resection and nothing for helping with rounds. So that's about $160. At that time, our overhead was running about 50 percent, so $160 would be $80. I was paying about 35 percent of my income in taxes; 65 percent of $80 is $52. The babysitter got $60 cash, so she took home more for sitting beside my pool and watching my kids than I did for four hours of medical work!

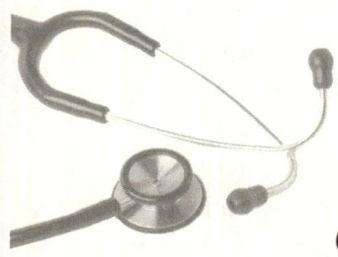

CHAPTER 8

DR. DEBAKEY STORIES

"When we want your opinion, we will give it to you." That was the policy about the opinions of residents who were in Dr. DeBakey's service.

I finished my training with a two-year residency with Dr. DeBakey at Baylor College of Medicine in Houston.

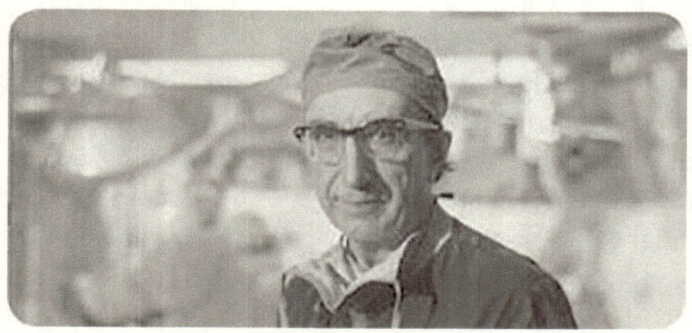

Michael DeBakey, MD

Here's a little background on Dr. DeBakey. He was born in August 1908. He grew up in Lake Charles, Louisiana. He did his residency at Tulane under a very famous surgeon, Dr. Alton Ochsner. He and Dr.

Ochsner made one of the earliest links between cigarette smoking and lung cancer. He is also credited with starting the mobile armed surgical hospital units (MASH units) during World War II. In the 1980s, he operated on the Shah of Iran. When I was in Houston, he was about seventy years old, and I was around thirty years old. He would get up at five in the morning, and it was difficult for me to get to the hospital earlier than he did. He was extremely impatient. When he was using an elevator, he would stand right in in front of the doors and go in or out as soon as they opened. If we had to wait too long for an elevator, his assistant had an elevator key and would call one of the elevators and tell the people on it that they had to get off because Dr. DeBakey needed the elevator.

His rounds were legendary. At around three o'clock in the afternoon, he would tell his assistant to call the consultants. About five or six cardiologists, a couple of neurologists and endocrinologists, and a smattering of other consultants would fill his office. The main attraction was watching him torture the surgical residents. The general surgery chief resident had to find all his X-rays and put them up in front of Dr. DeBakey in a very specific order. I had to do this job a few times when the general surgery residents were on vacation, and they took as much vacation from this rotation as they could.

The women in the X-ray file room would have to find the X-rays for the doctors because most of the time we were in the operating room right until the rounds started. So, we would come up and hope that the women had found all the X-rays. Like most workers in the United States, these women would generally feel that, if they found nine out of ten X-rays, they had done a pretty good job. However, Dr. DeBakey's opinion was a little different. When we got to the one X-ray that we didn't have, he would say things like, "See? I give you the simplest jobs, and you can't even do them! How can you expect to operate on my patients when you can't even find their X-rays?" Then he would ask, "Are you stupid or do you just not care?"

Fortunately, the Baylor residents told me the answer to that last one, the best answer was, "Lack of attention to detail, sir."

Another famous line Dr. DeBakey routinely threw at the residents at Baylor was "When we want your opinion, we will give it to you."

If somebody misfiled an X-ray and put it in another patient's envelope, it was gone forever. The smartest person in the world would not be able to find that X-ray. The great thing about the electronic systems, both the picture archiving and communication (PACS) and the electronic health records (when they are working), is that they can be accessed from pretty much anywhere. All you need is a computer with an internet connection, although it often is not easy to do from home at this stage of the game.

Another interesting story from my time in Texas with Dr. DeBakey is all about how our rotation in Saudi Arabia got started. Thoracic surgeons have to do a certain number of congenital heart operations as part of their residency, and more and more congenital heart operations were being done only at specific centers, usually one or two in each of the major cities. Before the Saudi Arabia rotation started, the Baylor residents would have to work with Dr. Denton Cooley, who had been at Baylor before his feud with Dr. DeBakey. They broke up over a disagreement about using artificial hearts. We would have to pretend we were on the pediatric surgical service at Texas Children's Hospital. We would actually go into the OR with Dr. Cooley so we would have a chance to participate in the requisite number of pediatric surgical congenital heart cases.

The Saudi Arabia rotation was great in numerous ways. First, it started in 1978 and lasted about ten years. I was there in 1980, the second year. We compiled our statistics for operations over the first two years during my rotation. We did mostly mitral and aortic valves, which was a great change from what we had done in the United States where 80 percent of open-heart surgery was coronary bypass surgery. But we also got to do congenital heart surgery on mostly young adults, which was easier than doing it on infants and toddlers. We did a lot of relatively simple operations like pulmonic valvotomies and atrial septal defect (ASD) repairs. The most complicated procedure I performed was to correct a Tetralogy of Fallot, a congenital heart defect that affects normal blood flow through the heart. Anything too complex was sent to a great surgeon, Magdi Yacoub, who was working in Egypt.

Another great thing about the rotation in Saudi Arabia was the amount of money that they paid us. I was making $17,000 a year as a seventh-year surgical resident in Houston, and when I went to Saudi Arabia, I was paid $12,000 a month as a junior cardiac surgeon. The senior cardiac surgeon was paid $1,000,000 a year. Unfortunately, Baylor had set it up so that the money went directly to Baylor, and Baylor paid the money to us, so Uncle Sam got to take about half the money as the 50 percent tax bracket started at $19,000 in those days. Still, it was a tremendous boon that enabled me to pay off my medical school loans, get a new car, and make a down payment on a condo when I came back and started work in New Jersey.

You may wonder how Dr. DeBakey negotiated such a great deal with the Saudis. In 1978, there were not a whole lot of heart surgeons making a million dollars a year in the United States. The way the story goes is that the Saudis asked Dr. DeBakey to set up this rotation, and he went to his surgical staff and told them that they wanted a proposal. The wives of the surgeons got wind of this, and they looked into how women were treated in Saudi Arabia at that time and decided that they definitely did not want to go to Saudi Arabia. However, they also did not want their husbands going to Saudi Arabia with a bunch of nurses for three or four months without them. So, they tried to put the kibosh on this whole rotation. The husbands just didn't say anything and hoped it would go away.

After a few months, at another staff meeting, Dr. DeBakey asked them what they had done about the Saudi proposal. They told Dr. DeBakey they really hadn't done anything, and he said, "Listen, the Saudis want an answer. You have to come up with something." The staff got together, and they came up with the bright idea that they would ask for so much money that the Saudis would turn it down. That is where they came up with the million dollars a year for the senior surgeon and $144,000 for the junior surgeon. What they didn't realize was that, like a lot of nouveau riche people, the Saudis would buy anything as long as it was expensive. At that time, they were pumping ten million barrels of oil a day at about $30 a barrel, and there were only six million Saudi Nationals and only about 5,000 members of the royal family among whom to divvy up the money that was coming out of the sand every day. One of the attending surgeons who went over there for six months made a half-million dollars. He said that rotation was "his ship coming in!" He put as much as possible in his pension plan.

One of the Filipino nurses who went to Arabia with us said, "Maybe if we prayed five times a day, they would find oil under the United States!" (Eventually they did—shale oil. It is just a lot harder to extract than the oil under Saudi Arabia.)

Probably the best thing about the rotation in Saudi Arabia was being exposed to the culture and meeting the people. My rotation was in early 1980 at a time when the hostages were still being held in Iran. We had also experienced the two Arab oil embargos of 1973 and 1978. The Arabs were getting a lot of bad press in the US at that time.

Meeting the Bedouins and seeing their culture gave us a totally different view. They were some of the simplest, most honest, and most religious people you could ever meet. My favorite memory was making rounds in the morning and seeing our patients sleeping on the floor with the sheets completely covering them. That was the way they had to sleep in the desert to keep the sand off themselves! They just were not used to sleeping indoors in beds.

Buying gas was another interesting experience. The oil embargos had driven gas prices way up in the US, but in Saudi it was dirt cheap! Also, the gas station attendants were not great at math, so rather than computing how many gallons you got times the cost per gallon, they had a simpler system. For small cars, they charged five riyals to fill up; for big cars, they charged ten riyals!

I have previously mentioned some of the difficulties that can occur during surgical residencies. I mentioned that, at Columbia Presbyterian, in my five-year general surgery residency, I was on either every other night or every third night. When we were on every other night, we worked approximately 120 hours a week. Every third came out to at least 100 hours a week. This was nothing compared to a few of the rotations at Baylor in Dr. DeBakey's residency where I did my thoracic and cardiac training.

Most of the residents were on every other or every third as I had been in my general surgery residency; however, there were two fellows who had rotations that were astounding even to me. One spent two months solid living at the hospital in a regular patient room. He was on call one hundred percent of the time for essentially two months. The only way he could get out was if the Baylor general surgery senior resident relieved him. This did not happen often for several reasons. One reason was that they had made a recent change in the rotation from three months to two months. Most of the senior residents had done this rotation for three months. They were often heard to say, "I'm not relieving him. I was stuck there for three months, and he's only in for two!" The other reason is that no one wanted to take the chance that Dr. DeBakey might come in and make rounds while someone was covering. If a doctor did not know everything about all his patients, someone would get fired.

Actually, this fellow was the luckier of the two. He was able to roam around the hospital. He could eat in the cafeteria. He basically had a private room even if it was just a hospital room. The other fellow was stuck in the intensive care unit (ICU) for two months. The ICU was huge, like everything in Texas. It had six bays of eight beds each and eight isolation rooms along the side. They used only seven isolation rooms because the ICU fellow lived in the other room.

This was a tiny room not much bigger than the bed. It was never quiet and never dark. Nurses could get in and call him at any time day or night. It was something like solitary confinement except they were confined *and* continually harassed. They were served meals just as if they were patients in the hospital. Needless to say, a few guys went a little bit crazy during this rotation. I came in one day and found one playing handball against the wall in one of the hospital corridors very early in the morning. I guess he just need to burn off some steam.

It was my job to relieve him. The same rules applied. As badly as he would like to get out of there, he would not want me to relieve him unless we were sure that Dr. DeBakey was at least out of Houston and preferably out of the country. Because, if Dr. DeBakey came in and found anything wrong with any of his patients, we would all be in a heap of trouble.

There was an entire network of people—starting with people who worked in Dr. DeBakey's office—whose job was to gather intelligence about when he was going to leave Houston. The entire hospital relaxed somewhat when he was gone, and it was during these periods that I could relieve the ICU resident. I think I relieved the ICU resident for three or four weekends in the four months I was on this rotation. The Baylor senior residents felt that I was way too lenient with them!

Approximately once a week, Dr. DeBakey would make what he called "full house rounds." He would also do these right before he went away and right after he came back from any major trip. He had been in the military and had helped develop the MASH units. His rounds were like a military operation. We rounded on approximately sixty patients distributed over ten floors of two hospitals.

We always took exactly the same path, same staircases. The head nurse of every unit would meet us at the door to that floor with the chart rack containing only Dr. DeBakey's charts. She would round with us. One or two of the younger residents would go out ahead of the rest as advance scouts. They would make sure that all the patients were in their rooms rather than in the bathroom or walking around the floor because their absence would slow Dr. DeBakey down. The residents would tell the patients, "Get into bed! Dr. DeBakey's coming!" There would be a lot of scurrying around and toilets flushing ahead of us.

One of the most famous Baylor stories comes out of this these rounds. I wasn't there when it happened, and it may just be an urban legend, but the staff at Baylor swore it was true. Supposedly Dr. DeBakey was making his full house rounds before he was going to leave the country to go to China for a few weeks. One of his patients in the ICU coded and died just before Dr. DeBakey was getting ready to make rounds. Now, you have to know that, when Dr. DeBakey rounded in the ICU, he didn't do a full physical exam on each patient. He stood at the foot of the bed, looked at the monitors, and checked the lab results. Mostly he listened to what the resident told him about the patient.

This particular resident must have been very resourceful. According to the story, he took the EKG leads and blood pressure cuff from the patient who had expired and put them on the (very-much alive!) patient in the next bed so that, at least on the monitor, the dead patient was exhibiting a fairly normal rhythm and blood pressure. As the story goes, as soon as Dr. DeBakey left the ICU, staff members called a code and pronounced the patient dead.

A lot of funny things happen on rounds. One of the funniest for me occurred when I was a young attending surgeon at Cooper Hospital in Camden, New Jersey, on an Easter Sunday in the late 1980s. I was making rounds, and the chief surgical resident was leading the group around. There were a few other residents and medical students—probably about five or six people in all. It was a beautiful day; the sun was shining, and all was right with the world. We went into a female patient's room. I don't remember her name, but I remember she was Polish, so I'll call her Ms. Kowalski. I had fixed a complex abdominal wall hernia about four days earlier. She was a heavy woman and had hardly been out of bed up to that point.

The chief resident was an excellent resident and eventually joined our group, but at that point, he was having some problems with the residency—something about his medical school transcript or something.

As the chief resident lead us into the room, we saw Ms. K running towards us with a look of fear on her face. She didn't even stop as we said hello. She went right to the bathroom. Initially we were happy to see her out of bed and moving around so well. Then we discovered the reason she was moving so fast—the chief resident stepped in a puddle of liquid human feces that was on the floor. We all almost died laughing!

However, the chief resident's life changed after that. His problems with the residency disappeared. He met a lovely girl; they are still married. He had a very successful career and, in fact, was the president of the New Jersey Medical Society for a year.

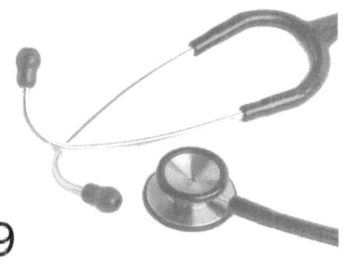

CHAPTER 9

SOME TECHNOLOGICAL ADVANCES

Hindsight is always 20/20.

I have mentioned some technological advances that have occurred during my career. A list of all of them would fill another book, but I will just highlight a few that I have been involved with over the years.

Pacemakers

I have always performed pacemaker implantation. I find them to be very interesting technologically. I have especially enjoyed watching them improve over the course of my career.

The first pacemakers were implanted back in 1950s. A man named Earl Bakken invented them in his garage in Minneapolis. His company later became Medtronic, which is now one of the largest health care corporations; they currently manufacture numerous different devices. The first implantable pacemaker was made by Medtronic in 1961.

The first time I heard about a pacemaker was when President Eisenhower had one implanted in the late 1950s. They had been around for a little while before that. Even when I went to medical school in the late 1960s and early 1970s, they were still pretty rudimentary. They were as large as a hockey puck, and the battery lasted only about two years. When I rotated on cardiac surgery at Massachusetts General Hospital in Boston in the spring of 1972, after the open-heart cases were finished, surgeons would replace two or three pacemaker batteries.

The two components of a pacemaker are the leads and the pulse generator. The pulse generator includes the battery and the electronics. Initially there was just one lead that went to the ventricle; the pulse generator was connected to this lead, and all it did was pace usually at seventy-two beats per minute. It did not try to read the patient's EKG, so was mostly used in patients with complete heart block. This also made them highly pacer dependent. After the patient was paced for several months, when the battery was changed, the patient would have no heartbeat until the new pulse generator was reconnected.

As the years went by, pacemakers got more and more sophisticated. The first innovation was the demand pacemaker. This was a pacemaker that monitored the electrical signals in the heart through the leads and paced only if the heart rate went below a certain number, which was usually set is either sixty or seventy. This was a great breakthrough as it's best to pace as little as possible.

Next came programmability. As I have mentioned, the original pacemakers were set at one rate. Around 1981, Medtronic developed a device that had a port sticking out the side so that surgeon could stick a needle through the skin into the port and adjust the pacemaker rate that way.

This got better and better; now, using radiofrequency, the pacemaker reps can change twenty parameters or more electronically without touching the pacemaker. Sometimes it can be done from thirty feet away.

This also made monitoring much better. Originally, patients had to have their pacemakers checked in the doctors' offices. Modems were a big breakthrough. Patients could call their doctors on the phone and hold the modem up to the phone. The doctor could read the rate remotely. When the rate dropped, that meant the battery was wearing out. Now most pacemakers come with a modem that sits by the patient's bed at night and is connected to the internet or a phone line. The modem checks the pacemaker every time the patient comes within thirty feet and can call in to a monitoring service if there any problems. The monitoring service contacts the cardiologist, who then contacts the patient. The next step will be a pacemaker that will send a patient an email that warns, "We have a problem!"

Rate responsiveness was another advance. These pacemakers contain a device that senses vibrations; they are apparently fairly common in the industry now. The device can tell how much a patient is moving around. Pacemakers that were set at a certain rate could not be adjusted for activity; in other words, even if a patient wanted to go up steps or perhaps have sexual intercourse or do any other type of exercise, his or her pacemaker was set at sixty or seventy or whatever rate at which it was programmed.

Activity monitors can deal with a range of heart rates. If a patient is sleeping, it will let the rate go down to the fifties. If the patient is running, going up steps, or doing some other vigorous physical activity, it will raise the rate to the nineties or higher as programmed.

The next step in the evolution was pacemakers with dual chambers. These pacemakers not only pace the ventricle but also the atrium.

In the beginning, we hated these because we found it very difficult to place the atrial lead. In the thirty or so years since they were developed, that has become easier, and now we put dual-chamber pacemakers in almost everyone except someone who is in chronic atrial fibrillation, which means that the atrial wall is just quivering and cannot be paced. Therefore, there's no point in placing a pacing wire.

In more recent times, biventricular pacemakers were developed. These not only pace the atrium and the right ventricle, but they also pace the left ventricle. This improves cardiac output and helps hold off on the development of atrial fibrillation and heart failure. Anyone with a low ejection fraction (a low cardiac output) who needs a pacemaker usually gets this type of device nowadays.

Here's a funny story relating to Medtronic. One evening, I was stuck at one of our hospitals with two patients who needed pacemakers. We started one at about five in the evening, and it went well. Then we started the second one at about an hour later. Right after we started, the image intensifier broke. This is the X-ray machine that produces "moving" X-rays," and we depended on it to see where the pacer lead was when we implanted it. There was a second machine available, so we waited while staff members brought that in—and then it broke!

It was going to take hours to get the repair crew in, so I decided to try to put the lead in with a normal X-ray machine, which took only static images. This was the type of machine that was used when we first started putting in pacemakers. We got the machine in, and within about fifteen minutes, we had the lead in excellent position and were done. We congratulated ourselves on how lucky we were.

The representative from Medtronic, who had been present for the procedure, had been wanting to go out for dinner at a brand-new racetrack that had just been built in the area. We figured this was the perfect time. We got there in time for the fifth race, and there was a horse running named Medatronic. We figured this was a message from God!

The horse was an eighteen-to-one longshot. We each put about $20 on him—a lot of money for us! He started off in first place, and we thought we were in for a big score. Slowly he started falling back until the announcer said, "He can see all the rest of them." He finished dead last. We did have a good dinner, and it was a beautiful facility.

Automatic Implantable Cardiac Defibrillators (AICDs)

Automatic implantable cardiac defibrillators (AICDs) are somewhat related to pacemakers, and most of them actually have pacemaker built in, but these are designed to shock the heart if the patient goes to ventricular fibrillation.

The first AICDs were developed by Dr. Michael Mirowski. He was born in Warsaw, Poland, and left his home at age fourteen to escape the Nazis. He was the only member of his family to survive the Holocaust.

The first implant of an AICD in a human was done in 1980. The first devices were huge, weighing nine ounces. They measured 8 x 11.5 centimeters. They were so big, we had to implant the device on the abdominal wall rather than the chest wall, which is where we implanted the smaller pacemakers. There were a lot of problems due to their size. Also, they had to be connected to two pads that looked like fly swatters. These were placed directly on the heart, usually via a thoracotomy (opening of the chest). The pads were just like the two pads that are placed on a patient's chest during a cardiac arrest when their hearts are defibrillated. The heart has to be between the two pads so the current can defibrillate it.

Because the pads are right on the heart, only low voltage is required. The external defibrillators usually start at 200 volts. They can go up to 1,000 volts. The AICDs typically deliver up to about 50 volts. In open-heart surgery, we could often defibrillate the heart with as little as 5 to 10 volts.

Because the AICDs were so bulky and because a thoracotomy was necessary to place the pads, only cardiothoracic surgeons could put them in. Also, the devices were rudimentary; for example, we had to place a magnet over them for thirty seconds to turn them on or off. When we turned them on, they would deliver a "test shock."

This led to a funny story about a patient who had an early AICD. He was moving, and he was loading his stereo system onto the truck. Back then, the speakers were often huge, and the woofer had a large magnet in it. So, he carried out the first speaker, and it turned off his AICD. Then he carried the second speaker, and it turned the AICD back on, and he got the test shock!

As time went on, the devices got much smaller and more sophisticated. A spring-like device that could be placed through a vein replaced the pads, so surgeons were no longer needed to place the device.

Now almost all the AICDs are placed transvenously by cardiologists who subspecialize in electrophysiology. This is just one of the many procedures that surgeons have done when they were new and difficult. Then other specialties took over when they got easier. A few other examples are arteriograms, which are now mostly done by radiologists or cardiologists.

Inferior vena cava (IVC) filters are devices that catch clots that develop in the legs and prevent them from getting to the lungs. Originally surgeons had to make an incision and "plicate" the vena cava, which is the largest vein in the body. When it got easy enough to do transvenously, the intervention radiologists took it over; that is, unless it comes up on a weekend or holiday. Then it usually goes back to surgery.

Most pacemakers are now placed by cardiologists specializing in electrophysiology.

Central lines are used to administer drugs directly into the heart; cardiac pressures can be measured at the same time. Initially they were placed almost exclusively by surgeons. Now many are placed by emergency room doctors or intensivists. Just five years ago, my surgical residents put in so many central lines that they were certified to place them alone in the first few months of residency. Now it can take years for them to get enough experience to do them solo.

Finally, as I have mentioned, coronary artery bypass surgery was the most common open-heart operation. Now about 80 percent of these procedures have been replaced by cardiac stents placed by invasive cardiologists through peripheral arteries. Furthermore, many cardiac valves are now being repaired or replaced by similar techniques.

Don't get me wrong—these changes have been great for our patients. They have just been tough on some of the surgeons. Dr. Wachter, in his book, *The Digital Doctor: Hope, Hype, and Harm at the Dawn of Medicine's Computer Age*, writes about the specialties that provide the most and least satisfaction for doctors. Cardiac surgery is listed as the least satisfying because "they train forever and then a lot of their work has been taken away."[2]

Also, expensive new technologies keep coming up. Fortunately, they work, but they also drive up the cost of health care. Even something as basic as wound care is involved. Here are several examples.

---

[2] Robert Watcher, *The Digital Doctor: Hope, Hype, and Harm at the Dawn of Medicine's Computer Age*

One new technology is vacuum-assisted wound closure (VAC). This is a simple system that works great. It involves cleaning out a large, chronic wound, most commonly a pressure ulcer, but it could be an abscess cavity or a surgical wound that dehisced (opened). The wound is cleaned, and a special type of sponge is applied. A suction device is then applied that contracts the sponge and pulls the wound together while draining off excess fluid. The procedure is usually repeated every other day. This has easily caused the healing of wounds that we were never able to heal in the past. The problem is that it is expensive. There are all kinds of payment systems for VAC, now but generally it runs about $60 a day. This may not sound like much, but that's $1,800 a month, and it often takes several months to heal a large wound. Also, there is the cost of labor for the physicians or nurses who are changing the dressing every other day.

One of my younger partners trained at Bellevue Hospital, one of New York City's best-known charity hospitals. Patients there often cannot afford VAC, so providers there they Gerry-rigged a system from materials they had on hand. They just moistened some gauze dressings with saline and put them in the wound. Then they covered the wound with a piece of Tegaderm, which is a medical version of a "press-and-seal "sheet. They made a small hole in this film and connected the wall suction. He said it worked great. I'm sure now the compliance officers will have a problem with this system!

If you think wound vacs are expensive, let me tell you about hyperbaric oxygen therapy, which involves using a decompression chamber for wound healing. When I learned to scuba dive, one of the things I had to memorize before each dive was the location of the nearest decompression chamber. The air in these chambers has a high oxygen content (for wounds it's 100 percent oxygen) at increased pressure of several atmospheres (for wounds it's usually 2 to 2.5 atmospheres).

Originally, these chambers were used by deep-sea divers for decompression sickness, also known as the bends, which occurs when a diver stays too deep for too long and then comes up too fast. The nitrogen in the bloodstream comes out of solution and forms bubbles. This can cause a lot of pain (hence "the bends"), but worse, if the bubbles get into the brain or heart arteries, they can cause a stroke or death.

For wound care, it has been shown that placing a patient with a chronic wound in such a chamber with 100 percent oxygen and 2 to 2.5 atmospheres of pressure every day for two hours promotes the healing of difficult refractory wounds. The problem is that it's very expensive. Medicare reimburses about $700 per treatment, but on average it takes about thirty-seven treatments to heal a wound, which adds up to $25,900 per wound. It has been shown that the medical costs of a nonhealing wound would be more than this. Because of the cost, its use is somewhat restricted. Generally, to qualify, a patient must have diabetes, osteomyelitis, or a history of radiation therapy to the involved area.

Expensive new therapies keep coming along. One intriguing one that is presently being evaluated is gene therapy for hemophilia A. This appears to work but is estimated to cost over one million dollars for a ten-year period! This sounds outrageous; however, in an article entitled "Gene Therapy for Hemophilia A: a cost-effectiveness analysis,"[3] the authors point out that the present treatment of uncomplicated hemophilia A is greater than $140,000 per year and that 30 percent of the patients develop inhibitors that drive the cost to over $1,000,000 per year. So gene therapy could be a relative bargain!

---

[3] N. MIchin et al., "Gene Therapy for Hemophilia A: a cost-effective analysis," *Blood Advances*, 2018 Jul 24;2 (14) 1792.

Extracorporeal Membrane Oxygenation (ECMO)

In most open-heart surgery, we use the cardiopulmonary bypass technique, which means a machine takes over the function of the heart and lungs while we stop the heart to repair it. This perfuses the rest of the body supplying oxygen to the tissues while the heart is stopped. This works well, but the longer a patient is on the bypass, the more likely it is that problems could occur, especially with coagulopathies, a condition that causes intractable bleeding after the bypass is removed. Any patient who is on cardiopulmonary bypass for more than four hours is likely to have problems when it is removed.

ECMO was first developed by John Gibbon and C. Walton Lillehei, both of whom were surgeons in the 1950s. Dr. Gibbon also performed the first successful open-heart procedure using the cardiopulmonary bypass technique. He repaired an atrial septal defect in an eighteen-year-old woman at Thomas Jefferson Hospital in Philadelphia on May 6, 1953. My first senior partner, Rudolph Camishion, was a medical student at the time and was present at that procedure. He complained a lot about how hard it was to clean that machine after each use. It had thousands of parts! A copy of the original device is on display at the Smithsonian.

ECMO was first used in neonates—babies who are four weeks old or younger—in 1965, and for the next thirty years, it was used primarily in children. In the last twenty years, it has been used more and more in adults. There was a tremendous increase in usage during the coronavirus pandemic in patients who developed severe pneumonia. If mechanical ventilation could not provide enough oxygen to the patient, ECMO treatment could be added. Usually, a cannula is placed in a vein to remove blood, which is then oxygenated through a membrane oxygenator. The oxygenated blood is then returned through another vein. There are many other uses for ECMO; for example, it is used during heart failure or a bridge to transplantation (maintaining the patient until a transplant is available). Most patients are weaned off ECMO after a few days; rarely, patients have remained on it for more than thirty days!

Obviously, this is a wonderful device, but it is difficult to imagine the cost of a thirty-day stay in an ICU on ECMO.

Robotic Surgery

The DaVinci Surgical System, developed by Intuitive Surgical, was approved by the U.S. Food and Drug Administration in 2000. The Women's Auxiliary at Cooper Hospital bought one for the operating room, and for a few years, it languished in a corner of the operating room as something of a plaything—like a video game. The consensus was that this was an amazing technology but was too cumbersome to actually use on patients.

Then, a few years later, the urologists gave it a try, and their regular use accelerated rapidly. According to an article in *Nature*, by 2009, 80 percent of prostatectomies were being done robotically. Subsequent studies showed no difference in overall results from robotic versus laparoscopic prostatectomies.

To me, this made sense because the robot uses laparoscopic tools and access sites. The only difference is that an extremely expensive robotic device is interfaced between the surgeon and the laparoscopic instruments.

The DaVinci robot costs around two million dollars, and the arms it uses run from about three to ten thousand. The arms must be replaced intermittently, which can increase costs from about three to ten thousand per procedure! This is a significant increase, especially when compared to the surgeon's Medicare reimbursement for common procedures like laparoscopic cholecystectomy ($683) or laparoscopic inguinal hernia repair ($546).

Robotic surgery is a very hot topic now. There are surgeons who love the robot and a growing number of surgeons, administrators, and lawyers who are having second thoughts about this technology.

Advantages include greater precision of movement than laparoscopic surgery, stereotactic three-dimensional visualization (there are two cameras a few millimeters apart), and access to difficult places like the pelvis and high up under the diaphragm. Additionally, some surgeons feel the process is more relaxing for them because they are seated a few meters away from the field at a console.

Disadvantages include, most significantly, cost! Other disadvantages are latency of movement of the arms (a slight delay as the computer moves the arms) and loss of proprioception (The robotic arms do not "feel"; in laparoscopic surgery, the surgeon holds the instrument and can feel how much pressure he is exerting.) Additionally, there is a steep learning curve. Indeed, many surgeons start doing simple procedure robotically so they will be more fluent with the robot when they have to do a complex procedure.

Many surgeons, at the moment, are in a bit of a quandary over surgical robots. I believe the robot is better for some complex procedures in difficult-to-access places like the pelvis; however, the average surgeon does not perform these complex procedures often. If he starts doing simple procedures robotically to improve his technique, he drastically ratchets up the cost of the procedure.

One of my best friends is a thoracic surgeon and chief of surgery at a hospital in South Jersey. When robotic surgery first started, he was very enthusiastic about it. He took the training and started doing chest procedures robotically. A year or so later, I asked him how he was doing with the robot. He said, "The hospital loses money every time I do a procedure with the robot. So, I stopped doing simple procedures with the robot. Then when a complex procedure came up, I was not comfortable using it."

I think that sums up the surgical robot situation.

My other reservation about using robots, at least for lung surgery, is that the surgeon is not scrubbed. He is sitting at a console a few meters away. I have done a lot of lung surgery, both open and thoracoscopically. No matter how careful a surgeon is, it has not been rare for a patient to experience significant bleeding, especially when the surgeon is working around the pulmonary arteries and veins for a lobectomy. Through an open thoracotomy, a surgeon can usually get a clamp on the bleeding very quickly. Even thoracoscopically, a surgeon is scrubbed, and the patient is prepped and draped. It usually takes only a few minutes to open the chest and stop the bleeding. In a robotic case, the surgeon has to first "dedock" the robot; in other words, disconnect the arms and back the robot from the patient. Then he must scrub, and someone has to prep and drape the patient. Then the surgeon must open the chest, find the bleeding vessel, and clamp it. I cannot see how all this can be accomplished in less than fifteen to twenty minutes. A patient can lose an awful lot of blood through a bleeding pulmonary artery in fifteen to twenty minutes!

To finish up this discussion, I will mention that an additional advantage to the robot is marketing. Many people feel this is the chief advantage just as cost is the chief disadvantage.

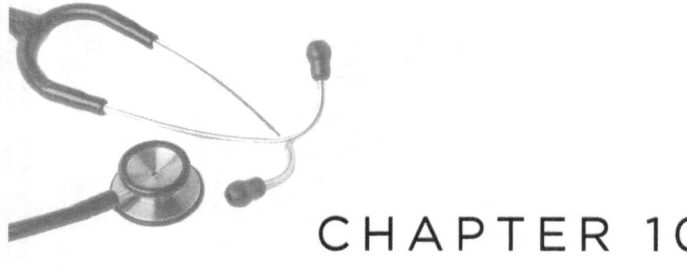

CHAPTER 10

EASY STEPS TO BETTER HEALTH FOR AMERICA

"You are what you eat."
All Americans have to do to improve their health is do less.

Diet

First, eat less, especially red meat and processed meats. I've read this advice in many places, most clearly in Dr. Michael Greger's excellent books *How Not to Die: Discover the Foods Scientifically Proven to Prevent and Reverse Disease* and *How Not to Diet: The Groundbreaking Science of Healthy, Permanent Weight Loss*. He claims that, by reducing our meat intake, we will all be a lot healthier. It's hard to believe, but he presents a lot of evidence that vegans are the healthiest people. I'm not ready to go vegan, but I have reduced the amount of meat in my diet.

One of the facts that made me believe this is that most anthropologists believe that humans did not routinely use fire for cooking until about 250,000 years ago. This means that, for about the first six million years of human evolution, we were primarily vegetarians. Logically, it would seem that our gastrointestinal tract and other systems were designed for a diet of primarily fruits and vegetables rather than meat protein.

One of the major points in Dr. Gregor's books and other books on diet is that we should be eating a lot more fruits, nuts, and vegetables, especially those with fiber content.

A fringe benefit of reducing the amount of meat that humans consume is that it would drastically reduce the amount of carbon dioxide and methane produced by the huge numbers of cattle and pigs on the planet. At first, I didn't believe this, but I keep reading about it in various sources and hearing about it in podcasts. An example is an article by Urvi A. Shah and Gia Merlo, "Personal and Planetary Health—The Connection With Dietary Choices," in *The Journal of the American Medical Association*. JAMA2023;329(21) 1823-24.[4]

So many of the animal species on the planet are nearly extinct or at least endangered, but there are three or four species that are doing just great. These are the ones that we've chosen to eat like beef cattle, chickens, and pigs. Their statistical numbers indicate they are thriving, but their lives are not so pleasant. They generally are kept in confined spaces and fed continuously until they are slaughtered. They are also given steroids and antibiotics and other drugs to fatten them up and control disease. There are a lot of medical concerns about what these chemicals do to us when we eat the meat. You know the old saying—you are what you eat.

My point is that simply eating less—especially less meat—would accomplish a lot of worthwhile goals simultaneously. People would

---

[4] Urvi A. Shah and Gia Merlo, "Personal and Planetary Health—The Connection With Dietary Choices," *The Journal of the American Medical Association*. JAMA2023;329(21) 1823–24.

lose weight, which would be a wonderful aid to good health. Fewer animals means that less carbon dioxide and methane would be produced, which would be a wonderful thing for the health of the planet. Also, there would be a lot more food available. It takes something like a hundred pounds of corn or other vegetables to produce every pound of beef. We could give that hundred pounds of food to the people on earth who are still going hungry.

The more I take care of sick people every day, the more I realize that most of America's health problems are self-inflicted. Alcohol, tobacco, drugs, and lack of exercise have made us one of the least healthy nations in the world. It's embarrassing to think about the image that people in Europe and the East have of us here in the United States. They see us as morbidly obese, lazy, materialistic people who do nothing but shop, eat, and exploit the rest of the world's population.

Alcohol

Alcohol has been around since the dawn of time. It's so easy to make that there's no way to keep humans from consuming it. Our ill-fated experiment with prohibition showed us that. A side effect was that we created a cash crop for organized crime.

When I did my four-month cardiac surgical rotation in Saudi Arabia—where alcohol was illegal—in 1980, the pump technicians had me hooked up with a still in less than a week. All the people there made their own wine and beer in closets in their apartments! The Saudis must have known what was going on because grape juice in bottles with resealable Mason jar–type lids were available in the markets. This airtight seal was needed to ferment beer or champagne. Also, in the stores, which had very little on the shelves, we could buy hops, an ingredient in beer making. I have never seen hops in a supermarket in America! People there could make beer or a decent white wine in a few weeks. A good red took a lot longer.

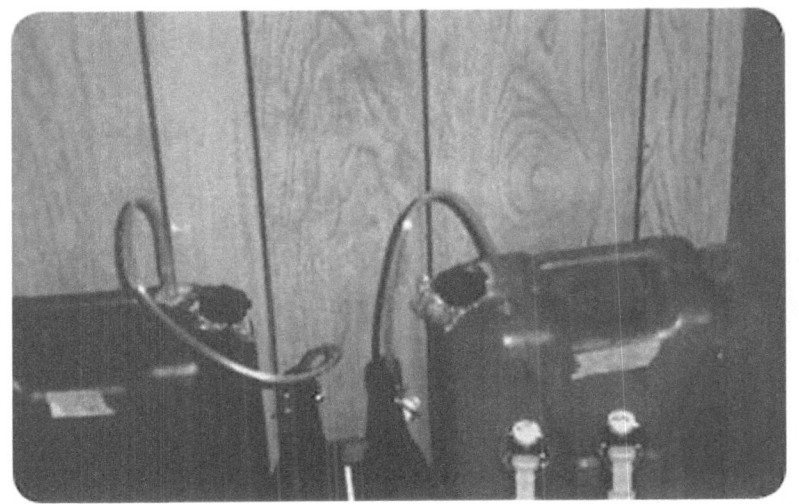

Author's still

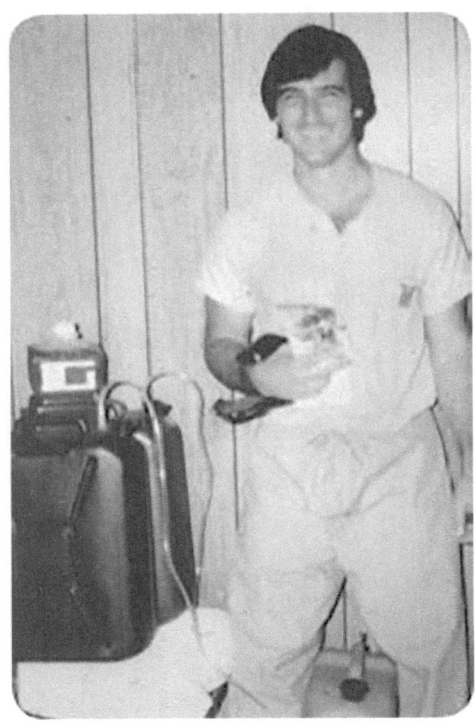

Author in still

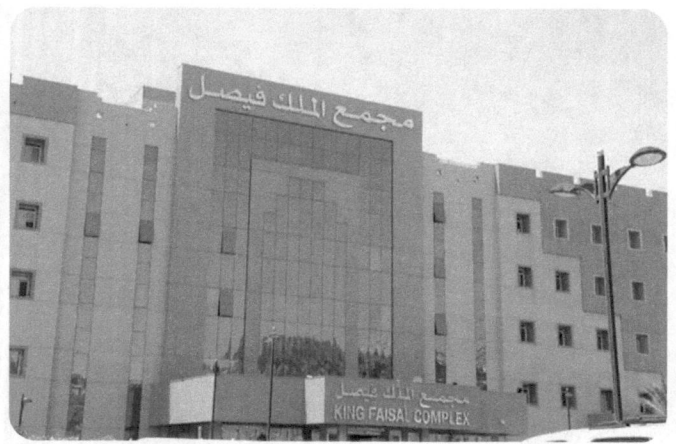

King Faisal Specialist Hospital in Riyadh, Saudi Arabia

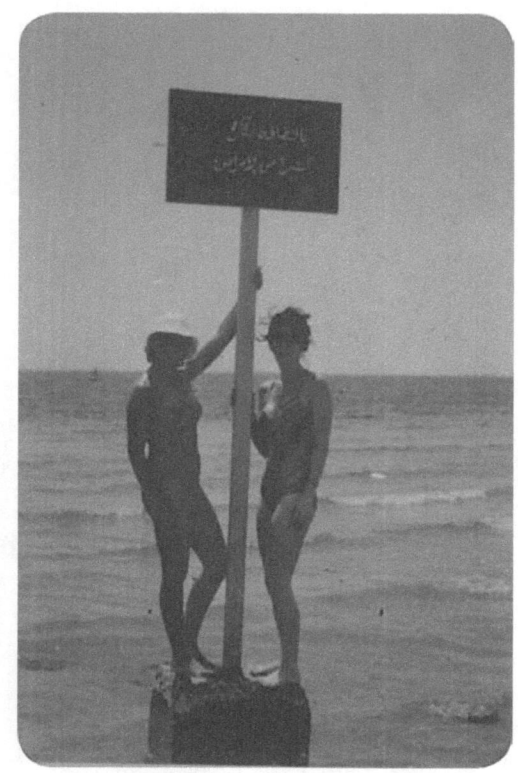

Beach in Dhahran, Saudi Arabia

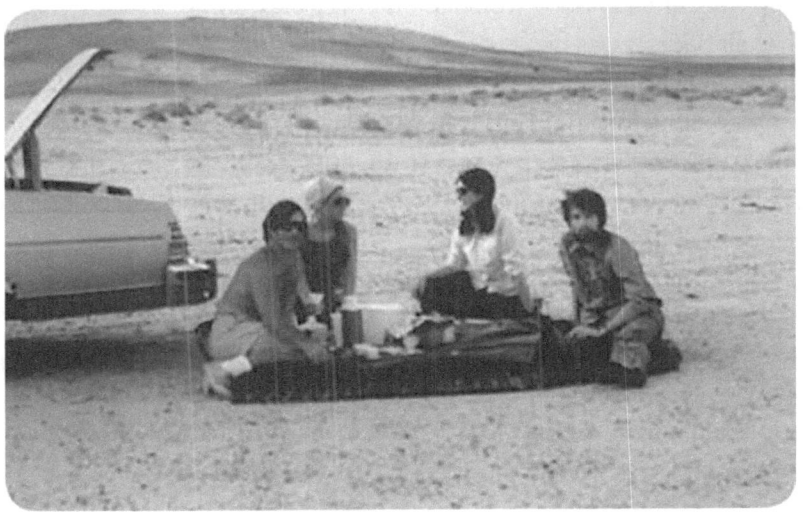

Picnic in Desert, Saudi Arabia, circa April 1980

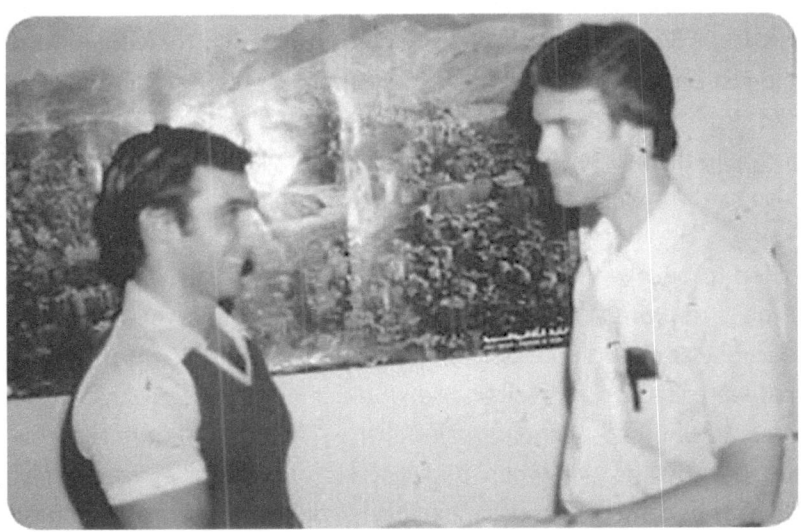

Happy moment- handing off the
beeper at the end of 7 years of residency

When residents were preparing to go on this rotation, the residents who were already there would ask them to pack some brewer's yeast in their bags; it was necessary for the production of good beer, and it was unavailable in Saudi Arabia. There was only one health food store in Houston that sold it at that time. After the Saudi rotation had run for a few years, a resident would go in the store and ask for brewer's yeast, and the clerk would say, "When are you going to Saudi Arabia?"

In the past, there was a lot of evidence that small amounts of alcohol were good for us. Most of the things I've read indicated up to about two ounces of alcohol per day actually prolongs life. That would be approximately two beers a day or two glasses of wine or one or two mixed drinks.

More recent studies, such as one published by Tim Naimi, MD, director of the University of Victoria's Canadian Substance Use Research in a recent JAMA Open Network study, have changed this. They found the risk of dying prematurely was 21 percent greater for women who had just under two drinks a day and 15 percent greater for men who had three drinks a day. Numerous other studies that I have come across in the last few years have come to similar conclusions. Some have said the best amount of alcohol is none at all.

I used to believe that a small amount of alcohol daily was good for us because, when I studied pathology at Dartmouth in the 1970s, our teacher was a tough old German pathologist. He did demonstrations that we called organ recitals. He would show us the organs of the patients who had been autopsied that week. I should note that this was back in the day when pathologists did autopsies frequently. This has become a rare event because an autopsy now costs at least $5,000. No one wants to pay for that unless they think there's some money to be gained from a lawsuit. The medical examiners also perform autopsies when foul play is suspected; however, routine autopsies are now almost never done in general hospitals.

In these organ recitals, the pathologist would show us the organs of alcoholics. Alcoholics tend to die at young ages. He would show us the livers, which were totally destroyed by cirrhosis and then show us aortas and arteries, which many times were as smooth as a baby's. There definitely seemed to be some protective effect of alcohol on atherosclerosis. However, even when a person exceeds the two-ounce limit, the negative effects of alcohol outweigh the advantages.

One of the most frustrating things is taking care of young alcoholics in the hospital. Most of them are males, and they tend to all look alike. They are disheveled and have scruffy beards and scraggly hair and large protuberant bellies often full of fluid called ascites. They come in, and we tune them up; then they go out and drink again until the next time they are admitted.

Tobacco

If we spent less money on tobacco, we would spend less money on health care due to tobacco-related illnesses. Lung cancer is still the largest cause of cancer deaths by far. More than twice as many people die of lung cancer yearly than of any other individual cancer even though we have made significant progress in reducing the smoking rate. About 18 percent of the adult population still smoke.

The new concern in this area now is electronic cigarettes, known as e-cigarettes, which emit a vapor that contains nicotine and other chemicals. The long-term effects are completely unknown as they've been around for only a decade or so. Most of the experts feel they are somewhat safer than regular cigarettes, but that has not been proven. Also, there is strong concern that young people who start off smoking e-cigarettes will eventually move on to smoking tobacco cigarettes.

A vast amount of money is spent yearly on tobacco in the United States and worldwide. This leads to vast amounts of money being spent on tobacco-related illnesses. Additional money is spent on litigation related to mesothelioma and other cancers. If you don't think that there's a lot of money to be made in this industry, all you have to do is watch late-night TV and see all the law practice commercials about mesothelioma.

People know about lung cancer and emphysema; however, smoking kills more people through heart disease and vascular disease. Atherosclerosis is a process that narrows the arteries all over the body. It does the most serious damage to the heart because, when the heart stops working, you die! However, most peripheral vascular disease resulting in claudication or pain on ambulation and eventually amputations are the result of smoking. Almost all aortic and most other aneurysms are the result of smoking.

Aside from lung cancer, smoking causes cancer in virtually every organ that the chemicals associated with smoking touch in the body. This includes cancer of the mouth, tongue, larynx, esophagus, stomach, kidneys, and bladder.

Nowadays, more and more studies are coming out that recommend lowering the amount of alcohol that is considered beneficial. Indeed, numerous studies now indicate that the best number is zero. It's hard to pin down what is responsible for this change. If I had to guess, I would say is because people are smoking less. Also, millions of people are on statin drugs now, which have lowered cholesterol and cut down on the incidence of heart disease. These beneficial effects may have wiped out the beneficial effects related to alcohol. This leaves only the non-beneficial effects of alcohol.

There is evidence that alcohol use leads to an earlier onset of dementia. Cigarette smoking also probably contributes to dementia. It seems obvious to me that most dementia is caused by vascular disease in the brain, so that anything that increases vascular disease in the brain is going to contribute to dementia.

Manual Labor

We should stop hiring people to do our menial tasks. I'm talking about mowing our lawns, cleaning our houses, and watching our children. By doing more of these sorts of tasks ourselves, we can achieve double savings. We could save the money that we would have to pay for the services and benefit from the increase in physical activity. Walking or jogging short distances as opposed to jumping in the car for a short drive could also help tremendously. A lot of current literature indicates that people who walk at work a few miles a day are much less likely to have heart disease and dementia than people whose jobs are totally sedentary.

Drugs

Another big improvement we could make in our lives is to take fewer drugs—and I mean legal drugs. Obviously, the main culprit here is the opioids, which can be addictive, but before we get to that, I would strongly suggest that the medical community and their patients consider trimming down polypharmacy in general.

As a surgeon, I write very few prescriptions other than short courses of opioids for postoperative pain and occasional short courses of antibiotics for pre or postoperative infections.

However, when we evaluate patients for surgery, we find that many of them are on more than ten prescription medications. When I was a resident at Columbia Presbyterian in the 1970s, we used to say no one should be on more than six pills a day. Now it feels as if everyone over the age of fifty is on more than six pills a day.

Diabetics used to be on insulin several times a day. Now they're often taking three or four different medications including several types of insulin. The new synthetic insulins are apparently much better for long-term therapy but also way more expensive than beef or pork insulin used to be.

The newer direct oral anticoagulants (DOACs) like Eliquis and Xarelto have largely replaced the older anticoagulants like warfarin (Coumadin). DOACs list at $388 to $566 per month. Warfarin costs $4 per month. Of course, there are advantages to the DOACs. They do not have to be monitored so closely with blood tests like warfarin does. On the other hand, there are disadvantages to DOACs. They cannot be monitored with simple blood tests. Also, there is a simple, cheap antidote to a warfarin overdose—vitamin K. For years there was no antidote for bleeding due to the DOACs; now there are several options such as Andexxa, but it costs $20,000 to 50,000 per dose! Because it is so expensive, most hospitals do not carry it in their pharmacies. It has to be ordered when a patient is bleeding, and it can be many hours before the medicine arrives.

People who have hypertension (high blood pressure) used to take one or at most two prescriptions, usually some type of beta blocker and a diuretic (water pill). Now it is not uncommon to see people on three to five different medications for hypertension. Most people over fifty take a statin to cut down on cholesterol. Many are on two or three more cardiac medications. Add to this vitamins, stool softeners, assorted supplements, sleep meds, pain meds, and various forms of anticoagulation drugs, and many adults are on more than ten pills a day. I've had patients on as many as twenty-three pills a day. No computer can calculate all the possible interactions between these many medications.

An article in the October 1, 2023, issue of the *Journal Demography*, which is published by Duke University, pointed out that Americans spend about half their lives on prescription drugs. The authors estimated that a boy born in 2019 will have a life expectancy of 76.59 years and will spend thirty-seven of those years (48 percent of his life) on prescription drugs. A girl will have a life expectancy of eighty-two years and be on prescription drugs for forty-eight years (60 percent of her life). The authors also discussed polypharmacy and pointed out that 42 percent of adults over sixty-five were taking five or more medications.

The authors specifically discussed the overuse of antibiotics, noting that there are five antibiotics prescribed for every six Americans every year. At least a third of these are unnecessary. This contributes to antibiotic resistance. More than 2.8 million infections occur in our country every year leading to about 35,00 deaths.

I think the biggest waste is on the dementia meds, which cost a fortune and have never been shown to have much effect. The FDA just granted accelerated approval to lecanemab for Alzheimer's disease. The data I've seen indicates that it doesn't cure Alzheimer's and will not improve memory or thinking. It has been shown to clear the amyloid plaques in the brain, and it is hoped that this will slow the progression of the disease in patients with early, mild Alzheimer's. Whether this will pan out or not remains to be seen. What is certain is that, since it was FDA approved, Medicare will start covering 80 percent of the cost. The cost is estimated to be $26,500 a year!

Another group of drugs of questionable value are the selective serotonin reuptake inhibitors (SSRIs) or anti-depression drugs. About 15 percent of Americans are on these drugs, which are very powerful and have a wide range of side effects. The problem I have with them is that many of the people who are depressed are depressed for a good reason. They have serious problems involving health, family, finances, work, and other life issues. I don't see how putting a Band-Aid on these problems by taking a pill is going to make them better. In fact, taking a pill that helps them ignore the problems is likely to lead to the problems getting even worse!

Of course, now everyone knows that the use of opioid pain medications has created a vast and growing problem; indeed, there are thousands of overdoses every day. I first became aware of this about ten years ago when an emergency medical technician told me that they used to carry with them about five or six doses of Narcan (generic name—naloxone), which is an antidote for opioid overdoses. He said they would often run out of it by noon. The opioid overdose situation has continued to get worse; in fact, it has continued to get worse throughout my entire career since I did my general surgery residency at Columbia Presbyterian in New York City, which was basically the capital of drug use at that time.

Living in New York City is like living in the future. Things always happen there first, especially if they are bad. Witness the coronavirus crisis in our present time. In the book *The Making of a Surgeon*, Dr. William Nolen wrote in 1970, "There will always be a drug addict coming into the emergency room with an abscess at 2 a.m. in the morning."[5] This has not changed. New York in the 1970s was a terrible place. I was one of the few graduates of Harvard Medical School who wanted to go there, and I wanted to go there only because my family was right across the Hudson River in North Jersey and the Yankees were right across the tiny East River in the Bronx. In fact, Columbia Presbyterian Hospital, where I worked, was built on the ground that the Yankees played on when they were called the New York

---

[5] Nolan, William. *The Making of a Surgeon.*

Highlanders. The area is called Washington Heights—get it? New York went through a terrible time in the 1970s. We had the Arab oil embargo in 1973, made worse by some terrible winters—one that was extremely cold, and one dumped about sixty inches of snow. To make things even worse, New York City went bankrupt in 1975 and had to close several hospitals. I happened to be working at Francis Delafield Hospital, which was right across the street from Columbia Presbyterian, when it closed. It is sad to see a hospital have to close.

Anyway, there were always drug addicts and there were always plans to control the drug problem, but in reality, somehow these plans always get delayed or diverted or just do not work. There are the infamous methadone maintenance clinics. These have created a cadre of methadone addicts who have to line up every day to get their daily methadone dose which, by the way, is an opioid just like heroin, Dilaudid (generic name—hydromorphone), and fentanyl. The only advantages are that the drug is taken by mouth and it blocks the use of other opioids. Supposedly this keeps the patient from seeking harder drugs; however, I often see patients nodded out on the methadone, and it seems to me that very few of them ever maintain any gainful employment. The programs don't try to wean the patients off methadone because they have found that when they do, the patients use the plan so they can get down to a low dose and then they can afford to go back on heroin or oxycodone again.

Also, no one wants any of these clinics in their neighborhood because of the undesirable clientele.

Other plans have been the War on Drugs, sponsored by the Drug Enforcement Administration (DEA) and the Bureau of Alcohol, Tobacco, Firearms and Explosives (ATF). This effort endeavors to take down drug cartels in Columbia, Mexico, and other places. This type of plan will never work because, the harder it is for people to get the drugs, the more the cartels will be able to charge for them.

It also ruins the lives of many honest American, Mexican, and Central American agents, police officers, and judges who try to control the drug use. And that happens because the cartels are winning this war. The only way to solve the drug problem in the United States is to curb the Americans' appetite for drugs.

I get a kick out of the nightly news when reports show viewers a huge cache of drugs that our agencies have intercepted—like an entire tractor trailer full! I always wonder how many of these tractor trailers are getting through.

Obesity

Lifestyle modification with regular exercise, even something as simple as walking, would be a lot cheaper and more pleasant way to maintain health overall.

Age and obesity turned out to be the two biggest predictors of mortality in the coronavirus pandemic.

No, we can't do much about aging; that happens to all of us every day. We can, however, treat obesity, and the best way is a sensible Mediterranean-type diet and regular exercise.

"Exercise is the Most Important Medicine for Covid-19" according to a review in *Current Sports Medicine Reports*.[6] Exactly how much exercise is a topic of much debate with a range from one hour a week in three twenty-minute sessions to up to eight hours a week. This is just what is necessary to remain healthy, not to train for a sporting event.

---

[6] Georgia Torres, Demitri Constantinou, Philippe Gradidge, et al, "Exercise is the Most Important Medicine for Covid-19," *Current Sports Medicine Reports* (CSMR.22(8):284-289, August 2023.

According to Professor Ralph Paffenberger, a pioneer in the field of physical activity physiology, "Everything that gets worse with age gets better with exercise." He is quoted in an article entitled "Association of Step Volume and Intensity with All-Cause Mortality in Older Women" in *The Journal of American Medical Association*.[7] This article establishes guidelines of 150 to 300 minutes a week of moderate intensity exercise like brisk walking or 75 to 150 minutes a week of vigorous exercise like jogging. It also suggests two sessions a week of muscle strengthening (resistance) exercises.

My exercise routines are largely Beachbody Workouts, which are an intense combination of aerobic and resistance exercises. I find that, if I do about three hours a week, I maintain fitness. At around five hours a week, I make some progress. When I can get myself to do eight to nine hours a week, I make much more rapid progress. That's just me; everyone is a bit different.

We all would be in better shape even if we just did the minimum three twenty-minute workouts a week as opposed to sitting on the sofa watching TV for another hour.

Walking is another underrated exercise. A great deal of research shows that people who have jobs that require walking live longer and experience much less dementia than people who sit at desks all day. One of the simplest tests for dementia is measuring walking speed. Most cellular phones have built-in pedometers that are fairly accurate. When I discovered this, I was surprised to find that I averaged walking three to four miles a day, most of it at work. I never would have guessed that just walking back and forth from the operating room to the patient floors would add up to that much!

---

[7]   I-Min Lee, Eric Shiroma, Masamitsu Kamada, et al., "Association of Step Volume and Intensity with All-Cause Mortality in Older Women," *The Journal of American Medical Association* 11/14/23 Vol 330 #18, 1733–4.

I am working in a wound care center now. About 50 percent of the problems I see are directly related to obesity. Pressure ulcers, venous ulcers, fungal rashes, and a host of other problems are all related to just being too heavy. Also, the heavier we get, the harder it is to exercise, so the heavier we get, and so on!

Probably another 40 percent of the patients I see are from various developmental centers. These are institutions that take care of the chronically ill. Many of the patients I see were born with cerebral palsy of other conditions that cause developmental delay. Many of them have been totally cared for their entire lives. Many of them are in their sixties and seventies.

They say a society will be judged on how it treats the poor, weak, and disabled. We are going to get high marks on this score! It is tremendously expensive and is one of the reasons we pay so much for health care in America.

The Edwin Smith papyrus, an ancient Egyptian medical text, was discovered in 1858. It describes the treatment of wounds that the Egyptians used in 1600 BCE! It is amazing how much they knew. In many ways, they were ahead of medieval medical practices. I am proud of cardiac surgery when I think about 5,000 years from now when the archeologists of the future will be looking at what we accomplished. When they see the remains of people with beautiful little artificial heart valves in place, they will have to think "These guys were pretty good!" We surgeons have already been upstaged by the cardiologists and device manufacturers who have figured out a way to place heart valves through an artery without the sternotomy incision. Where's the glory in that?

The United States spends an average of $12,914 per person per year on health care. Other similar developed countries spend $ 6,125—less than half as much. They get similar and sometimes better results.

We give by far the most vaccines to our children in the first five years of their lives, yet we do not have the healthiest kids. Junk food and lack of exercise contribute to this problem.

The official maternal mortality in America for 2021 was just published. It is discussed in an article in the October 2023 issue of *The Journal of the American Medical Association*.[8] The rate is 32.9 maternal deaths per 100,000 births, which is the highest rate since 1964. The US rate, even accounting for coronavirus-related cases, remains higher than the rate in any other high-income country. The National Vital Statistics System provided the data used in this article.

Bariatric Surgery and Obesity Medications

The latest wrinkle in the treatment of obesity is drugs like Ozempic and Wegovy (the generic name of both drugs is semaglutide), which started out as medications for diabetes. It was discovered that, as a side effect, many patients lost significant weight, sometimes 15 percent in a year or so. This was very desirable, especially since most diabetic medications up to then caused diabetics to gain weight, which made their diabetes worse.

Now many physicians are prescribing these drugs "off label" to non-diabetics along with other competing diabetes meds like tirzepatide and liraglutide for weight loss. Significant weight loss has been documented, but this is a relatively new use for these drugs, and experts are concerned about possible long-term effects. Often it takes years and tens of thousands of uses to sort out these issues.

An article in *The Journal of the American Medical Association* entitled "Continued Treatment with Tirzepatide for Maintenance of Weight

---

[8] Diana W Bianchi, Janine A Clayton, and Shannon Zenk, "Addressing the Public Health Crisis of Maternal Mortality," JAMA October 13, 2023 (doi:10.1001/jama.2023.19945).

Reduction in Adults With Obesity: The SURMOUNT-4 Randomized Clinical Trial"[9] described a study that followed 670 adults who took ten or fifteen milligrams of tirzepatide subcutaneously weekly for thirty-six weeks. They lost an average of 20.9 percent of their body weight! However, a subgroup received placebo from week thirty-six to week eighty-eight, and they regained 14 percent of their body weight. The overall weight loss for the group that continued on tirzepatide for eighty-eight weeks was 25.3 percent of body weight. Overall, at eighty-eight weeks, the group that was switched to placebo at thirty-six weeks lost 9.9 percent of body weight.

Prior to the arrival of these drugs, bariatric surgery was a common way to treat morbid obesity, and it still is. I have never done these operations, but I have taken care of hundreds of patients who have had these procedures, often when they came into the emergency room with complications.

For full disclosure, I have to admit that my feelings about bariatric surgery were colored by an early experience. Just a few months into my internship at Columbia Presbyterian, I was called to assist on a "cut down" to place a central line so we could give total parenteral nutrition to an eighteen-year-old girl who weighed over three hundred pounds and had gone into hepatic (liver) failure after a jejunoileal bypass. The seeming absurdity of having to pump calories intravenously into a three-hundred-pound woman never left me!

Jejunoileal bypass was the popular bariatric procedure in the 1970s. It was abandoned shortly thereafter because of serious complications. Turns out it's not a great idea to bypass most of the small intestine! Since then, numerous other bariatric procedures have come and gone.

---

[9] Louis Aronne, Naveed Sattar, Deborah Horn, Harold Bays, et al., "Continued Treatment with Tirzepatide for Maintenance of Weight Reduction in Adults With Obesity: The SURMOUNT-4 Randomized Clinical Trial," JAMA online on December 11, 2023(doi10.101/jama2023.24945).

As I said, my feelings are colored by this experience. Also, I always felt that this was a surgical solution to a behavioral problem. Finally, there is a basic surgical principal—never disturb normal anatomy unless you have a very good reason to do so.

Currently, bariatric surgery has gotten much better. The advent of laparoscopy was a huge breakthrough for bariatric procedures. Now they can be done through three to five trocar (a medical device) sites each less than one centimeter. Previously, surgeons were required to make a midline incision. In a person with a body mass index (BMI) of thirty-five or more (normal is around twenty-five) there are a lot of problems just from the incision, and these often lead to complications and even death.

Currently, the two common bariatric procedures are the gastric bypass and the gastric sleeve. Gastric bypass is more complicated, but it does generally lead to more rapid weight loss. Since it is more complicated, it leads to more complications. The gastric sleeve is a much simpler procedure. It just removes most of the lower part of the stomach—the greater curvature. A similar operation, a gastrectomy, has been done for cancer and ulcer disease for over one hundred years. After surgery, the stomach pouch is smaller so the patient feels full sooner and loses weight. We used to tell the gastrectomy patients that they would probably lose about thirty pounds.

Transgenderism
Primum non nocere.

The last modality I want to discuss is transgenderism. I thought long and hard about including this in my book because I don't want to create any more controversy on this topic. Also, please note that I am not speaking about homosexuality at all. That is an entirely different topic.

CHARLES ANTINORI MD, FACS

As a physician and a bit of a scientist, I feel obligated to point out that it is impossible to change a male to a female or vice versa. I am appalled by the fact that so many intelligent people are afraid to speak up on this topic, which is so cut and dried.

A pair of sex chromosomes, in humans and other mammals, determines the sex of an individual. It is a fact that 99.95 percent of humans have either XX chromosomes (females) or XY chromosomes (males). That's it—end of story! Our bodies have trillions of cells. Every cell in a male's body has XY chromosomes. Every cell in a female's body has XX chromosomes. This is biology 101!

I see my share of plastic surgery. I almost went into plastic surgery, but I am telling you that no plastic surgeon and no number of hormones can change a male to a female or vice versa.

No one even tried to do this for the first six million years of human history! When I was in medical school, we learned about the tiny percentage of people who now fall under the term *intersex*. Often, they are born with "ambiguous genitalia." Many times, this is due to some type of chromosomal abnormality. Geneticists look up the history of a given abnormality and try to figure out if the patient would do better as a male or a female. Then the surgeons—usually urologists, gynecologists, or plastic surgeons—get involved and try to match the genitalia to whatever sex is being assigned. Endocrinologists can also get involved with hormonal treatments. This was the start of what is now known as gender assignment surgery, and it should have been the end of it.

I'm not a psychiatrist, so I am not going to say that there is no such thing as gender dysphoria, but if a person is unhappy about his or her gender, I think trying to change it just makes things worse aside from the fact that it is impossible. This reminds me of when I was a resident. We often saw people who tried to commit suicide by drinking lye such as Drano drain cleaner. I felt sorry for these people because, no matter what problem they had before, they had just added a big one—not being able to eat normally for the rest of their lives. I don't see this form of suicide very often anymore. I think the word got out it this was an inefficient way to commit suicide.

All major sports have outlawed performance enhancing drugs (PEDs). Most of these are male hormones that make the male athletes into supermen in some regards. They get stronger and faster, but there are terrible side effects. And there are issues of unfairness in using a substance to change competitive balance.

Barry Bonds, who hit the most home runs in Major League baseball history, is not in the Hall of Fame because he was linked to PEDs. Roger Clemens, a pitcher who won a record seven Cy Young Awards is not in the Hall of Fame for the same reason.

PEDs cause acne, baldness, liver damage, bony abnormalities, and worst of all, increased aggressiveness or "roid rage." And that's just the result of taking androgens, an increased dose of male hormones. Imagine the consequences of females taking male hormones or males taking female hormones. This is unphysiological. Part of the "manifesto" of the female transitioning to male who committed the mass shooting in Nashville was just leaked. One must wonder how much the hormones affected her/his crazed ideation.

I have spoken about the overuse of drugs. Taking hormones, to me, is probably the worst use of drugs—a healthy male taking pills to change himself into an unhealthy female, or a healthy female taking pills to change herself into an unhealthy male. By the way, cosmetic surgery does not work either. The best plastic surgeon in the world can't turn a vagina into a fully functioning penis or a penis into a fully functioning vagina. They can just make something that looks something like a penis or vagina.

The plastic surgeons at Oregon Health and Science University (OHSU) feel that they are becoming very well known for genital surgery. Two operations that they are performing are phalloplasty, which is the creation of a penis, and a very popular procedure, robot assisted vaginoplasty, the construction or reconstruction of the vagina.

OHSU warns of complications with the vaginoplasty such as wound separation, tissue necrosis, graft failure, urine spraying, hematoma, blood clots, vaginal stenosis (narrowing), rectal injury, fistula formation, and fecal accidents.

Patients stay in the hospital for five days for wound care and catheter maintenance. Once home, they must continue the transgender hormones and manually dilate the "neo-vagina" in perpetuity to prevent the cavity from closing down.

The procedure is described in a handbook published by OHSU: "Surgeons first cut off the head of the penis and remove the testicles. Then they turn the penile-scrotal skin inside out and together with abdominal cavity tissue fashion it into a crude artificial vagina." The robotic arms are placed through trocars around the umbilicus (bellybutton) and the lateral abdominal walls.[10]

It would be difficult to stop adults from transitioning, especially if they have the financial resources to pay for it out of pocket; however, the current trend of leading six- and eight-year-olds down this path is insane. Puberty blockers are likely to cause permanent damage even if the person decides to "detransition" later in life. Right now, this seems to have become something of a fad with the younger generation. If you get bored with TV, the internet, social media, et al., just try transitioning. It makes you an instant celebrity. This fad can do a lot more damage than the hula hoop or disco dancing.

---

[10] Adapted from C.F. Rufo's opinion column in The Epoch Times 11/15-20/2023.

One of the major arguments in favor of transitioning is the supposedly high incidence of suicide in children who experience gender dysphoria. It is not easy to obtain solid facts on this subject because it is a relatively new phenomenon and is so emotionally charged. However, I have read that the suicide rate is very high after transitioning. Also, an unknown number of people change their minds and detransition.

I shouldn't even have to mention how unfair it is to allow fully grown males to compete in women's sports or allow men who are transitioning into women's locker rooms and bathrooms. I would have you just google "Riley Gaines" to hear her stories about how this has affected competitive women's swimming.

From a medical point of view, it has made a simple one-line question on an admission sheet—"Check one: male or female"— into a complicated issue that can fill a page and change overnight!

The most basic rule in medicine going back to Hippocrates is *primum non nocere*—"first, do no harm." One of the primary rules of surgery is never disturb normal anatomy. Transgender medicine and surgery violate both these rules.

I don't want people marching on my front lawn because of this statement. I just feel obligated to raise my voice to try to help people by steering them away from this crazy fad, which is bound to end badly.

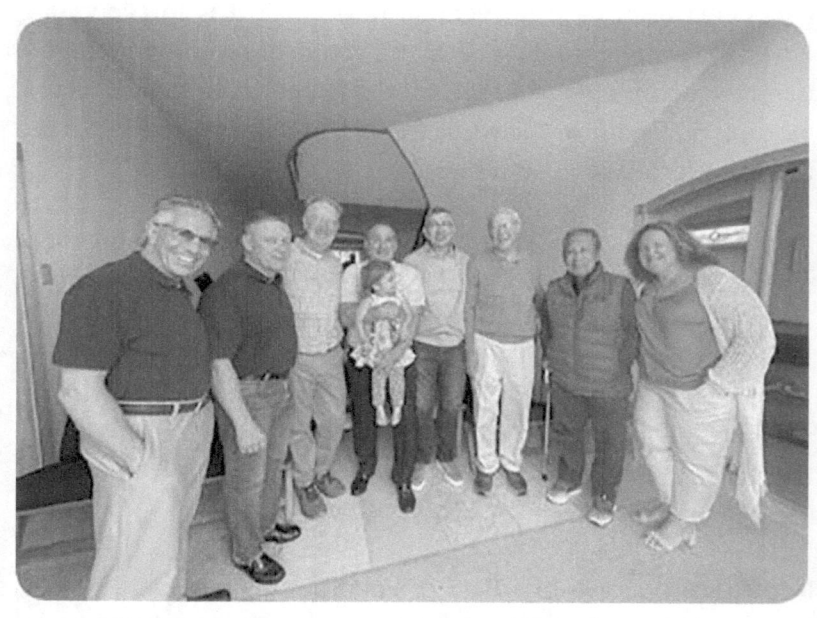

Surprise retirement party in May 2023. They said it was my granddaughter's (pictured) second birthday party.

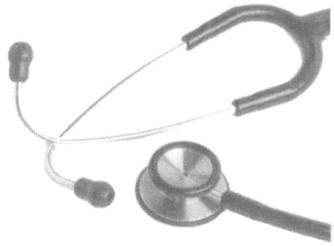

EPILOGUE

This is the first book I have ever written, although I have authored and coauthored a few dozen scientific papers. Overall, it has been an interesting if somewhat tedious project. I hope my readers will enjoy the book and gain a better understanding of health and health care.

If present trends continue, I think we are in for some difficult times in health care. The coronavirus debacle may have been just the tip of the iceberg. Many physicians and nurses feel the system is being held together with duct tape and rubber bands. Importing eight million indigent aliens is not likely to help the situation. I am amused by the nightly news reporting that "sanctuary cities" like New York and Philadelphia are reeling under the stress of a few thousand immigrants. What did they think was going to happen?

However, I think with some of the relatively minor modifications made to the health care system, things could get a lot better. All we have to do is *do less*.

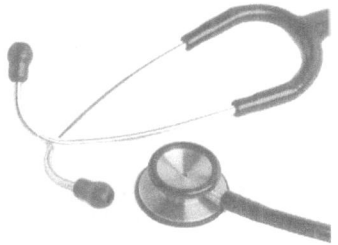

BIBLIOGRAPHY

Arndt, Brian, John W. Beasley, Michelle D. Watkinson, Jonathan L. Temte, Wen-Jan Tuan, Christine A. Sinsky and Valerie J. Gilchrist. "Tethered to the HER: Primary Care Physician Workload Assessment Using HER Event Log Data and Time-Motion Observations." The Annals of Family Medicine September 2017, 15 (5) 419-426; DOI: HTTPS://DOI. ORG/10.1370/afm.2121.

Aronne, Louis, Naveed Sattar, Deborah Horn, Harold Bays, et al. "Continued Treatment with Tirzepatide for Maintenance of Weight Reduction in Adults With Obesity: The SURMOUNT-4 Randomized Clinical Trial." JAMA online on December 11, 2023(doi10.101/jama2023.24945).

Bianchi, Diana, Janine A Clayton, and Shannon Zenk. "Addressing the Public Health Crisis of Maternal Mortality." JAMA October 13, 2023 (dci:10.100`/jama.2023.19945).

Dallas, Kai, Paige Kuhlman, Karyn Eilber, Victoria Scott, Jennifer Anger, and Polina Reyblat. "MP04-20 Rates Of Psychiatric Emergencies Before And After Gender Affirming Surgery." https://doi.org/10.1097/JU.0000000000001971.20

Greger, Michael, MD, and Gene Stone, MD. *How Not to Die: Discover the Foods Scientifically Proven to Prevent and Reverse Disease.* MacMillan Audio, 2016.

Greger, Michael, MD, and Gene Stone, MD. *How Not to Diet: The Groundbreaking Science of Healthy, Permanent Weight Loss.* MacMillan Audio, 2019.

Kennedy, Robert F. Jr. *The Real Anthony Fauci: Bill Gates, Big Pharma, and the Global War on Democracy and Public Health.*

Krauthammer, Charles, MD. *Things That Matter.* Random House Audio, 2013.

Lee, I-Min, Eric Shiroma, Masamitsu Kamada, et al. "Association of Step Volume and Intensity with All-Cause Mortality in Older Women." *The Journal of American Medical Association* 11/14/23 Vol 330 #18, 1733–4.

MIchin, N. et al., "Gene Therapy for Hemophilia A: a cost-effective analysis." *Blood Advances*, 2018 Jul 24;2 (14) 1792.

Makary, Marty, MD. *The Price We Pay: What Broke American Health Care—and How to Fix It.* (New York, Bloomsbury Publishing, 2019).

Nolen, William. *The Making of a Surgeon.* Mid List Press (1970, 1990) ISBN.922811-46-6.

Robert Wachter, Robert. *The Digital Doctor: Hope, Hype, and Harm at the Dawn of Medicine's Computer Age.*

Shah, Urvi A., and Gia Merlo. "Personal and Planetary Health— The Connection With Dietary Choices." *The Journal of the American Medical Association.* JAMA2023;329(21) 1823-24.

Sinsky, C., L. Colligan, L. Li, M. Prgomet, S. Reynolds, L. Goeders, J. Westbrook, M. Tutty, G. Blike. "Allocation of Physician Time in Ambulatory Practice: A Time and Motion Study in 4 Specialties." Ann Intern Med. 2016 Dec 6; 165(11); 753-760. doi: 10.7326/M16-0961. Epub 2016 Sep 6. PMID: 27595430.

Torres, Georgia, Demitri Constantinou, Philippe Gradidge, et al., "Exercise is the Most Important Medicine for Covid-19." *Current Sports Medicine Reports* (CSMR.22(8):284–289 (August 2023).

Wachter, Robert. *The Digital Doctor: Hope, Hype, and Harm at the Dawn of Medicine's Computer Age.* Whisper sync for Voice-Ready, 2015.

www.ingramcontent.com/pod-product-compliance
Lightning Source LLC
LaVergne TN
LVHW091531070526
838199LV00001B/20